SOMERSIZE
COCKTAILS

SOMERSIZE COCKTAILS

SUZANNE SOMERS

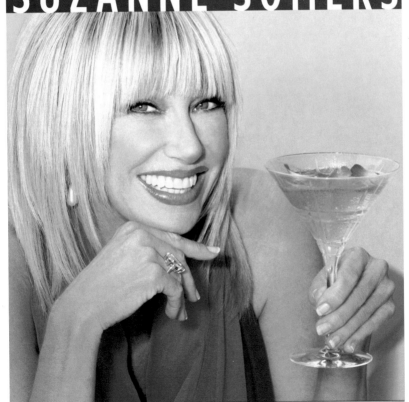

30

Sexy

Libations

from Cool

Classics

to Unique

Concoctions

CROWN PUBLISHERS, NEW YORK

Library of Congress Cataloging-in-Publication Data
Somers, Suzanne
    Somersize cocktails : 30 sexy libations from cool classics to unique concoctions /
Suzanne Somers.
    Includes index.
    1. Cocktails.   2. Low-carbohydrate diet—Recipes.   3. Sugar-free diet—Recipes.   I. Title.
TX951.S63   2005
641.8'74—dc22   2005015379

ISBN-13: 978-1-4000-5330-8
ISBN-10: 1-4000-5330-7

Printed in the United States of America

Design by Lauren Dong

10   9   8   7   6   5   4   3   2   1

First Edition

To my dad, Ducky: You taught me everything I need to know about alcohol and drinking responsibly.

Contents

Acknowledgments   8

Introduction   10

SOMERSIZE MOJITO   17

MANGO MOJITO   19

WATERMELON MOJITO   21

POMEGRANATE MOJITO   23

BLENDED CITRUS LAVENDER SMOOTHIE   25

RUBY RED GREYHOUND   27

LEMON DROP   29

CANDY CANE HOT COCOA   31

COSMOSA   33

DIRTY JALAPEÑO MARTINI   35

JUNGLE JUICE   37

THE BERRY CHOCOLATE MARTINI   39

LONG ISLAND ICED TEA   41

BLOOD ORANGE SCREWDRIVER   43

WATERMELON DAIQUIRI   45

IRISH COFFEE   47

FRESH APPLE MARTINI   49

TANGERINE POMEGRANATE FIZZ   51

PIÑA COLADA   53

CARAMEL APPLE MARTINI   55

SANGRIA   57

STRAWBERRY FIZZ   59

MINT JULEP   61

LYCHEE MARTINI   63

SPICED CINNAMON MOCHA   65

FRESH LIME MARGARITA   67

COSMOPOLITAN   69

CHOCOLATE ESPRESSO MARTINI   71

MANDARIN ORANGE MARTINI   73

GINGER LIME COOLER   75

Accessories Guide   76

Index   80

Acknowledgments

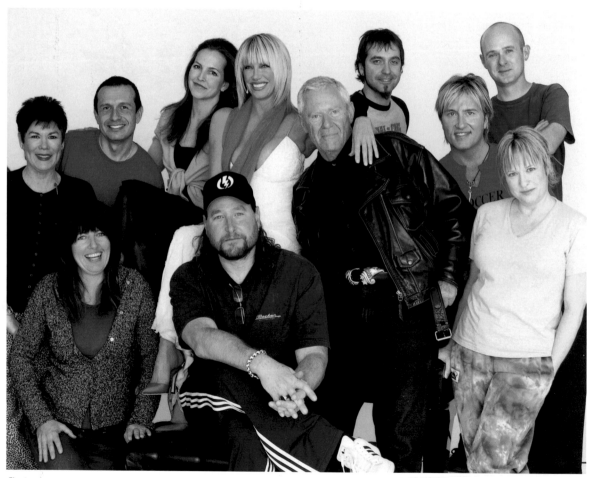

The team.

As with all my Somersize books, Caroline Somers was my right arm, left arm, and legs. You are invaluable to me. Your integrity regarding the Somersize program insures that we never get off track. Your palette is the best this side of Italy. Your intelligence, enthusiasm, and your beautiful soul are all a source of inspiration to me. Thank you for your continuing support, and for being the best daughter-in-law ever, the most wonderful mother to my grandchildren, and an incredible wife to my son, Bruce. You are a keeper and I love you.

To Kenny Pyle, mixologist to the stars! You taught me so much about cocktails and how to incorporate all my favorite flavors into delicious drinks. Thanks for making every detail just right. Also thank you for creating my Somersize Drink Mixes. No one else could get them to taste as great as you have. And thanks to my dear friend, Garry Kief, for introducing us.

To my photographer, Jeff Katz, we really had fun on this one. The cover was magic and the drink shots are innovative and simply gorgeous. Thanks to your fabulous team, Jack Coyier, Victor Boghossian, Gabriel Hutchison, Andy Strauss, and Stuart Gow.

Thank you to my food stylists and special effects team of Denise Vivaldo and Cindie Flannigan of Food Fanatics. I had no idea what a science project this would be. It was fascinating and you made everything look luscious!

To my prop stylist, Laurie Baer, and her team of Claire Harbo and Katie Hofsomer, thank you for finding so many interesting surfaces and backgrounds as well as the fabulous glassware. Stunning!

Thank you to Mooney on hair. You know every strand so well by now!

To Barbara Farman on makeup, thank you for making me shine without the shine.

Thank you to Xavier Cabrera on wardrobe for pulling together a great look.

To Marsha Yanchuck for more awesome proofreading. To Julie Turkel, for making sure I'm exactly where I'm supposed to be, and to my assistant, Liz Kozakowski, for bringing the stores to me when I can't get out.

Special thanks to my editor, Lindsey Moore. You did such a great job while Kristin Kiser was out on maternity leave. If Kristin wants a sibling for her daughter, I know I'll be in good hands with Lindsey!

Thank you to my greatest supporters at Crown—Jenny Frost, Steve Ross, Philip Patrick, Tina Constable, and Tammy Blake. More thanks to the production team—Amy Boorstein, Trisha Howell, Leta Evanthes, and Lauren Dong. To Dan Rembert, who did the cover design, this may be my favorite one yet.

Thank you to my attorney, Marc Chamlin, for keeping it legal.

To my literary agent, Al Lowman, I raise my glass to you in heaven.

And to my husband, Alan Hamel, we've been toasting one another for thirty-five years and it's just the beginning.

Thank you to each and every one of you. I couldn't have done it without you. Cheers!

Introduction

What is it that is so sexy about a perfect cocktail? And why is it so mesmerizing to watch a good bartender create scintillating potions? Although I rarely drink hard alcohol, one great cocktail really kicks off a special evening. Even if I don't finish it, I enjoy the experience of holding a beautiful glass and taking small sips from a frosty drink.

I love to entertain, and the cocktail hour sets the tone for the evening to come. On New Year's Eve I might serve champagne in beautiful flutes lined in rows on a tray to say, "You are in for an elegant evening." On the other hand, a pitcher of margaritas says, "You are in for some casual fun." A martini bar sets a sexy tone. Having these wonderful recipes for interesting cocktails or non-alcoholic beverages enhances that mood. It's all part of the entertaining details that make for a great event.

Cocktails have made a major comeback in the past decade. Gone are the days of the plain martini, when the only variation was how dry you liked it. I never understood those drinks because I don't like the taste of hard alcohol. I always felt cocktails were for serious drinkers. And because I have alcoholism in my family, I steered clear. While I usually stick with an occasional glass of wine, I have recently been introduced to some fabulous, fanciful cocktails. These are in no way the type of drinks that serious drinkers prefer. These are the kind of drinks in which the taste of the alcohol is usually masked. Some might call them "sissy drinks" but I just call them fresh, exotic, and delicious. In most cases, these drinks can be made without alcohol and are just as appealing.

This is a book of cocktails that will set a tone for your meals. I have used all of my favorite flavors, such as mint, lemon, lime, tangerine, ginger, grapefruit, pomegranate, watermelon, and even chocolate, to name a few. You'll find a few classics, but even those are imbued with a twist. After all, who needs a recipe for a screwdriver or a greyhound, but make it a Blood Orange Screwdriver and a Ruby Red Greyhound and it's a whole new world.

Just as I do in my Somersize books, I suggest you use the highest-quality ingredients for these recipes. From the quality of the alcohol to the quality of the mixers to the taste of the ice (old ice can ruin a drink)—it all matters in making a perfect drink. Each recipe is made from scratch, with alternative shortcuts using my Somersize Cocktail Mixers and other products from my line that are made without refined sugars (all available at SuzanneSomers.com).

For those of you on the Somersize program, you may be wondering how alcohol fits in, since it remains on the forbidden "Funky Food" list. Many types of alcohol do not contain carbohydrates, including vodka, gin, rum, brandy, and whiskey. While they contain no carbohydrates, your body will still burn this alcohol as fuel before it will burn off your fat reserves as fuel. With this knowledge, these spirits have been recently ranked as Almost Level One, meaning that if you are doing well on your Somersize program and steadily losing weight, you may enjoy them in moderation. Tequila is generally cut with 50 percent sugar water and contains 99 carbohydrates for 1½ ounces; however, 100-percent agave tequila has no carbohydrates. Agave is the highest-quality tequila and the only type I recommend you have while on the Somersize program. Other alcohols to stay away from are flavored alcohols. Many of these are made with sugar and flavorings that are usually used to mask a less expensive product.

Although no one can confirm the exact time-frame, most historians agree that the word *cocktail* dates back to the early nineteenth century. Every country takes credit for remarkable inventions. As Americans, we are known for baseball and apple pie, but did you know that the cocktail was also born in the United States? During the jazz age in the 1920s, the cocktail became extremely popular. This was also the time of Prohibition, and because alcohol was banned, many people started making their own. Since the bathtub versions or smuggled illegal brands didn't taste very good, other ingredients were added and the cocktail came into vogue. At the time, bartenders didn't have the variety of mixers that are available to us now. Just walk into any nice restaurant or bar and you will be wowed by the creativity on the drink list.

There is a myth that cocktails are hard to make—but they really aren't. All you need are a few simple tools: a metal shaker, a shot glass, a stirrer or bar spoon, a muddler (a wooden stick to grind fresh herbs or fruit), and an array of beautiful glasses. In this book you will see references to several types of glasses:

A martini glass is easily recognizable with a long stem and broad cone-shaped glass.

The margarita glass (sometimes called a *cocktail glass*) is similar to the martini glass, but it has a rounded bowl. Drinks that call for these glasses can also be served in martini glasses.

A highball is a tall, thin glass that usually holds cold drinks, often served with straws.

The old-fashioned glass (or rocks glass) is a short, squatty glass for alcohols served over ice or without a lot of mixer.

Wine glasses are generally stemmed with an open bowl.

Champagne flutes are long and narrow with an elegant stem.

No matter what the style, I always prefer thin glass. I don't like drinking from thick glass, especially for delicate drinks.

As for garnishes, this is really where you can make your drinks special. We've all seen the typical mint sprig, lime wedge, and maraschino cherry hundreds of times. Get creative with orchids, rose petals, cactus wedges, and more. Find interesting ways to cut fruits and vegetables and skewer them on unique drink stirrers. This is the fun part and will really tell your guests that every detail is important.

Another essential element of your cocktail hour is the appetizers you choose to serve. I have written a whole book of delicious recipes, *Somersize Appetizers,* to go beautifully with your Somersize cocktails. Imagine a balmy summer night that begins with a Lemon Drop accompanied by Grilled Scallops Wrapped in Prosciutto with Basil-Parsley Pistou. Host a lovely ladies' luncheon with the pink, delicate Cosmosa sparkling in your prettiest champagne flutes, served with Artichoke Bottoms with Dungeness Crab Salad. Get together with old friends for a cocktail party of Dirty Jalapeño Martinis served alongside Mini Burgers with Gorgonzola and Caramelized Onions. Let your exotic side show with a Lychee Martini paired with Tuna Tartare with Chili-Ginger Vinaigrette on Pappadam Chips. Get in touch with Asian influences by starting an event with a Mandarin Orange Martini and Seared Tuna with Cilantro-Orange Sauce. Or have the whole family over for a Sunday brunch that begins with a Strawberry Fizz and my Somer Frittata. These are knockout combinations!

Although I have many favorites in this book, if I had to pick one it would be the mojito. In fact, I am so enjoying this drink that I have given you four variations on this traditional lime-and-mint creation. All you do is combine fresh mint leaves, lots of squeezed Key lime (yes, the flavor is much better than that of regular Persian limes), SomerSweet (or sugar), and crushed ice with a splash of soda water. Traditionally, a mojito is "muddled." In this process the sugar is ground into the mint leaves and helps to release the mint oil. I have found that when using SomerSweet in place of sugar, it's more effective to shake the ingredients vigorously in a shaker since the SomerSweet doesn't grind into the mint leaves in the same manner as the sugar. I simply add the lime juice with peels, fresh mint, SomerSweet, vodka or rum, and crushed ice into a shaker. Shake until well chilled and pour the contents, including the lime peels and mint leaves, into a highball glass. Add a splash of soda water and you are ready to impress your guests.

In Cuba, this drink is served with rum. I usually drink it sans alcohol, but when I do include alcohol, I prefer vodka because it is tasteless. My husband, Alan, prefers rum, so we offer our guests their choice. An icy cold mojito with the mint leaves and squeezed lime right in the glass is cool and refreshing and just a delight. For an island twist, try the Mango Mojito (so good!) with my Chili-Braised Pork with Tomatillo Salsa. Check out the Watermelon Mojito paired with my Summer Salad on a Skewer. Or the Pomegranate Mojito with Curried Lamb Skewers with Mint-Cilantro Chili Paste. Divine combinations!

I hope you have as much fun with these recipes as I had creating them. If you are drinking alcohol, responsibility is paramount. Do not get behind the wheel of a car and do not let any of your guests drive if they are intoxicated in any way. In fact, the testing of these recipes took place at the home of my son, Bruce, and Caroline's house (my daughter-in-law who works by my side on these books). Alan and I had our assistant join us so that she could drive us home. Caroline was already at home and did not have to worry about driving anywhere. We tasted about ten drinks over the course of three hours. Just a sip of each was enough. At the end of our day, none of us were even tipsy. When my granddaughter came home from school she was not feeling well. Caroline needed to take her to the doctor, but would not drive herself. She asked a friend to drive them (in Bruce's brand new car) just to be safe. The friend promptly pulled out of the driveway and smashed the bumper of the car against a brick pillar—and she hadn't been drinking at all! A bit of irony, but the point is to be responsible. The costs are much too high.

That being said, let the cocktail hour begin! Have fun creating romantic, exciting, sexy, or casual fun parties with these varied and delicious creations. Your guests will feel so very special and you will be the toast of the town!

Enjoy,

SUZANNE SOMERS

SOMERSIZE COCKTAILS

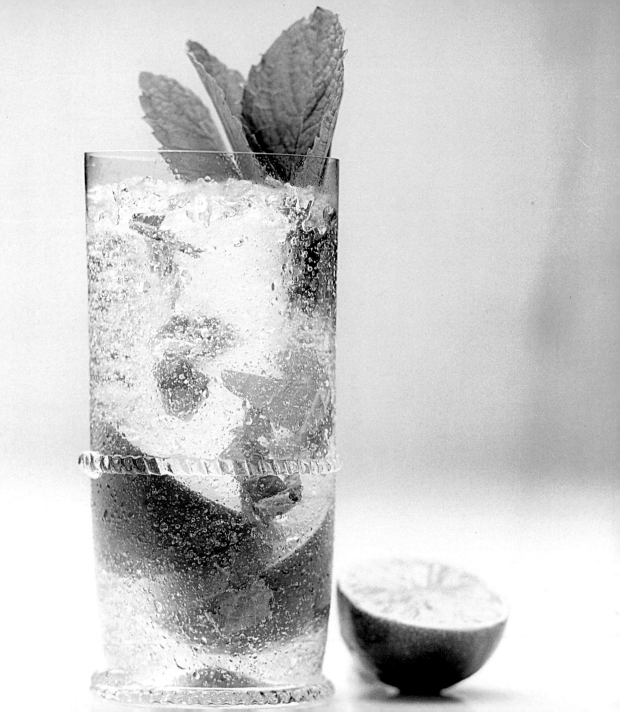

SOMERSIZE MOJITO

SERVES 1

This Cuban drink is light and refreshing, with a burst of fresh mint and lime. Normally it's sweetened with sugar, but I use SomerSweet instead. I have to say, I actually like the taste of SomerSweet better! Sugar can leave a bubbly film in your mouth but SomerSweet is so clean and fresh tasting. Traditionally this drink is made with rum, but I much prefer the taste of vodka. Make it whichever way you like. This is the perfect summer drink. There are many different preferences when it comes to mojitos. I tend to like mine with strong lime and mint flavor. Some like it less intense with more club soda. Adjust to your liking. This is also delicious without any alcohol.

To a cocktail shaker, add the rum, mint leaves, lime juice (with squeezed lime peel), SomerSweet, and ice. Shake vigorously for 15 to 20 seconds to release the fresh mint flavor. Pour the contents, including the mint leaves and lime peel, into a highball glass. Top with a splash of soda water and gently stir to combine. Garnish with a mint sprig.

2 ounces light rum or vodka

6 to 8 fresh mint leaves

Juice from 1 1/2 Key limes (or 1/2 regular Persian lime), plus lime peel

3/4 teaspoon SomerSweet (or 1 tablespoon sugar)

About 3/4 cup crushed ice (large handful)

1 ounce soda water

Mint sprig, for garnish

Somersize Product Version

Place the Somersize Mojito Mix, rum, and mint leaves into a cocktail shaker. Shake vigorously for 15 to 20 seconds to release the mint flavor. Serve in a highball glass over ice and top off with the soda water. Gently stir to combine. Garnish with a mint sprig.

2 ounces Somersize Mojito Mix

2 ounces light rum or vodka

2 mint leaves (or more)

About 3/4 cup crushed ice (large handful)

1 ounce soda water

Mint sprig, for garnish

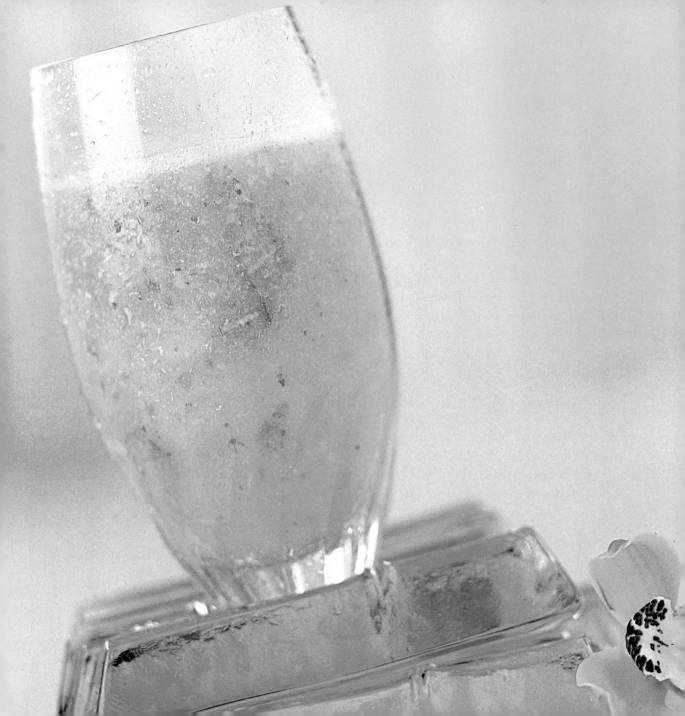

MANGO MOJITO

SERVES 1

Oh, my! This drink is reason enough to have a party. Virgin, with vodka, or with rum, this one will transport you to a tropical island.

To a cocktail shaker, add the vodka, mint leaves, mango chunks, SomerSweet, and ice. Shake vigorously for 15 to 20 seconds to extract the mango juice from the fruit and release the fresh mint flavor. Add the soda water and pour the contents, including the mango chunks and mint leaves, into a highball glass.

2 ounces vodka or light rum

6 to 8 fresh mint leaves

$1/4$ cup fresh mango chunks (1-inch cubes)

$1/2$ teaspoon SomerSweet (or 2 teaspoons sugar)

About $3/4$ cup crushed ice (large handful)

1 ounce soda water

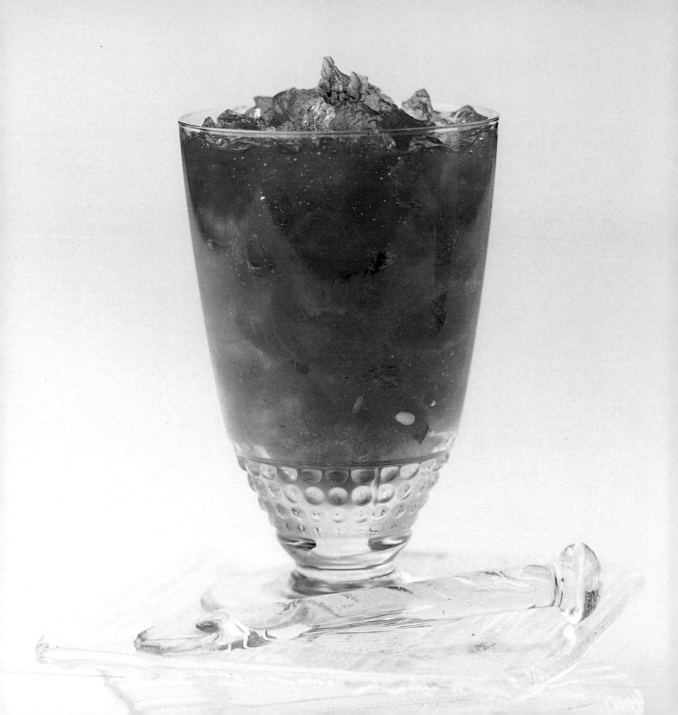

WATERMELON MOJITO

SERVES 1

My husband, Alan, *loves* watermelon, so I made up this recipe for him. In the heat of summer, nothing hits the spot like a ripe, juicy watermelon. Here I've added it to my favorite mojito, and it sings! It can be made without alcohol for a fruity watermelon cooler. The added sweetener or sugar is optional depending upon the sweetness of the melon.

To a cocktail shaker, add the vodka, mint leaves, watermelon chunks, Somer-Sweet, lime juice, and ice. Shake vigorously for 15 to 20 seconds to extract the watermelon juice from the fruit and release the fresh mint flavor. Add the soda water and pour the contents, including the watermelon chunks and mint leaves, into a highball glass.

2 ounces vodka or light rum
6 to 8 fresh mint leaves
$1/4$ cup fresh watermelon
   chunks (1-inch cubes)
$1/2$ teaspoon SomerSweet
   (or 2 teaspoons sugar)
Juice from $1/2$ Key lime
   (or $1/4$ regular Persian lime)
About $3/4$ cup crushed ice
   (large handful)
1 ounce soda water

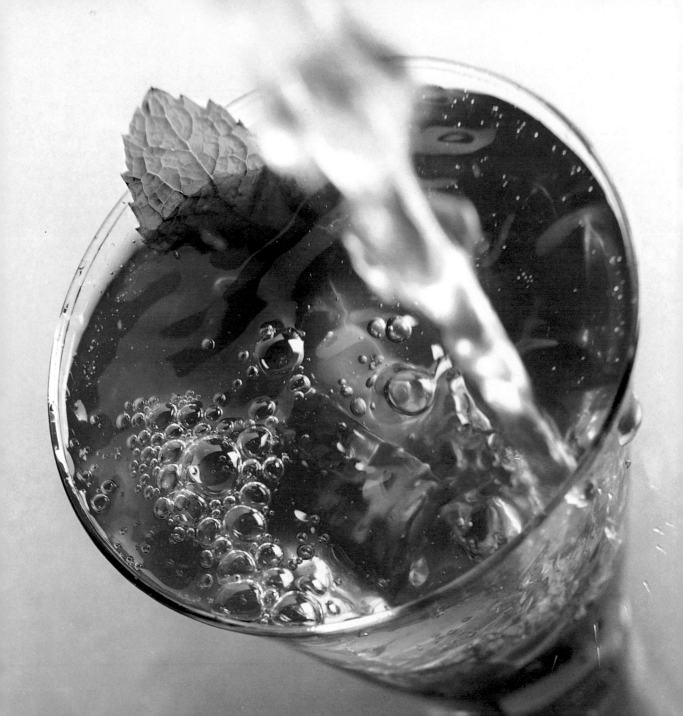

POMEGRANATE MOJITO

SERVES 1

Up the winding stone steps to my home I have a 30-year-old pomegranate tree. It bears fruit twice a year, in April and October. I make lots of wonderful things with the pomegranate seeds and juice. This drink is my ode to the pomegranate. Omit the vodka for a refreshing nonalcoholic drink.

To a cocktail shaker, add the vodka, mint leaves, pomegranate juice, Somer-Sweet, lime juice, and ice. Shake vigorously for 15 to 20 seconds to release the fresh mint flavor. Add the soda water and pour the entire contents into a highball glass. Garnish with a sprig of mint and a few pomegranate seeds.

2 ounces vodka or light rum

6 to 8 fresh mint leaves

2 ounces unsweetened
   pomegranate juice

1/2 teaspoon SomerSweet
   (or 2 teaspoons sugar)

Juice from 1/2 Key lime
   (or 1/4 regular Persian lime)

About 3/4 cup crushed ice
   (large handful)

1 ounce soda water

Mint sprig, for garnish

Pomegranate seeds, for
   garnish

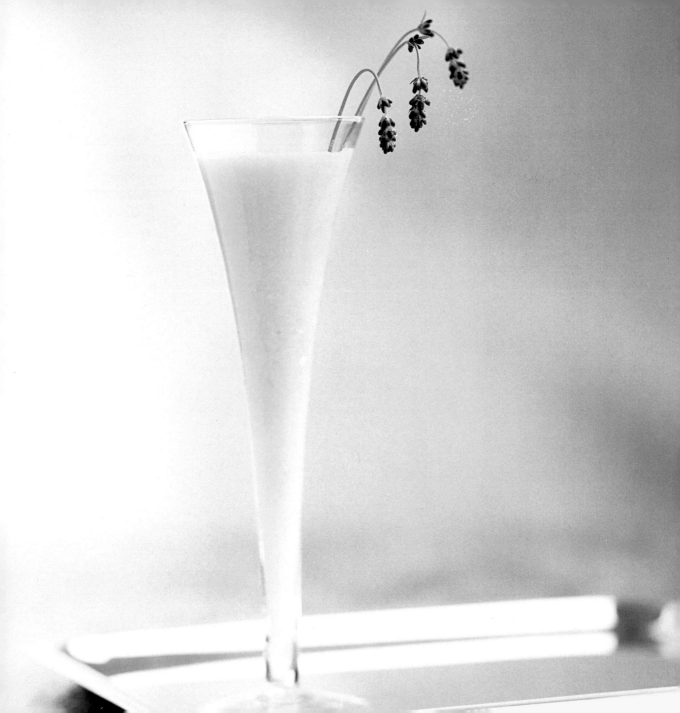

BLENDED CITRUS LAVENDER SMOOTHIE

LEVEL TWO

SERVES 2

This drink was created from the many types of citrus we grow in the desert. I use whatever we have on hand: Meyer lemon, lime, grapefruit, orange, or tangerine. I usually make it without alcohol, but it's great either way. This drink is so ethereal, I call it the drink they give you when you arrive in heaven.

Make a simple syrup by heating 1 cup water and the SomerSweet in a saucepan over high heat until the SomerSweet dissolves completely. Add the lavender sprigs and lower the heat. Let the lavender steep in the simple syrup for at least 30 minutes. Remove from the heat, strain, and cool in the refrigerator.

Place the citrus juice, ½ cup (4 ounces) of the lavender simple syrup, and ice into a blender. Blend until smooth. Pour into highball glasses or fancy champagne flutes and garnish with a sprig of fresh lavender.

---

4 teaspoons SomerSweet (or ½ cup sugar)

3 lavender sprigs, fresh or dried

3 ounces vodka, gin, or light rum

2 cups freshly squeezed citrus juice (any combination of Meyer lemon, lime, grapefruit, orange, or tangerine)

Ice

Sprig of fresh lavender, for garnish

25

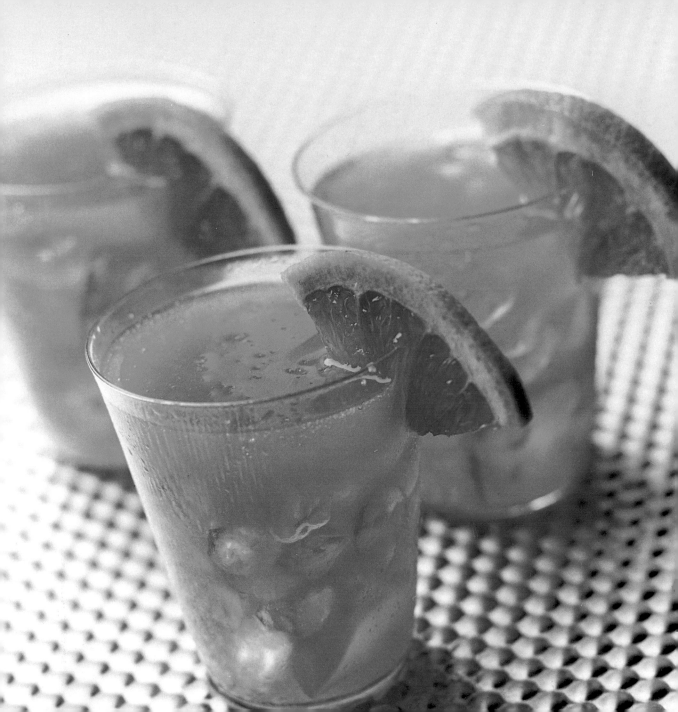

RUBY RED GREYHOUND

SERVES 1

The desert is citrus heaven. Some of my most prolific trees are Ruby Red grapefruits, and they are one of the most delicious God-given tastes. Here it is combined with vodka to take this classic drink to a new level. Just like in your cooking, the quality of your ingredients makes all the difference in your drinks.

Place the vodka, grapefruit juice, and SomerSweet into a cocktail shaker with ice and mix thoroughly. Pour the entire contents into an old-fashioned or highball glass and garnish with a Ruby Red grapefruit wedge.

$1\frac{1}{2}$ ounces vodka

4 ounces Ruby Red grapefruit juice, preferably freshly squeezed

$\frac{1}{2}$ teaspoon SomerSweet (or 2 teaspoons sugar), depending upon the sweetness of the juice

Ruby Red grapefruit wedge, for garnish

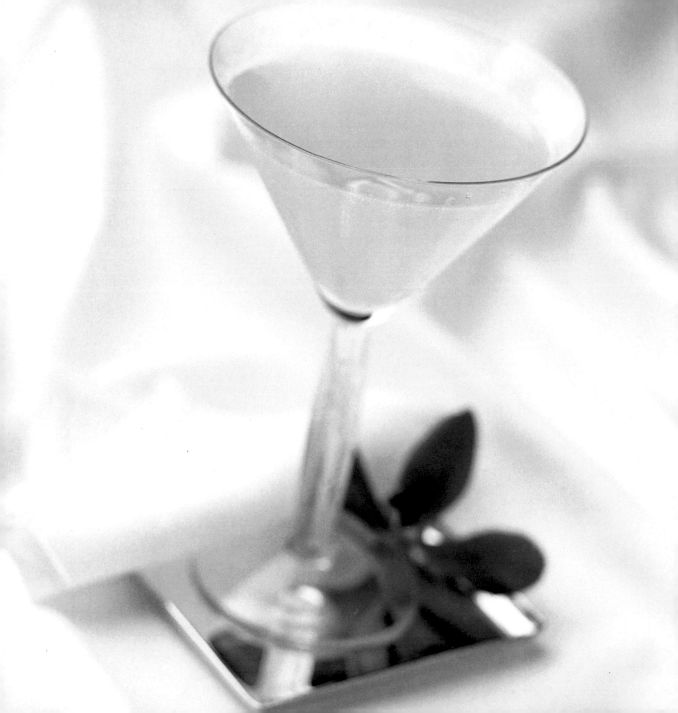

LEMON DROP

SERVES 1

The lemon tree in our desert home covers the front patio outside the kitchen. When the lemons drip from the boughs we make lemon everything . . . including the cleanest, freshest drink around, a Lemon Drop. It's like lemonade for adults. If you don't feel like squeezing fresh juice, take a shortcut and use my Somersize Margarita Mix.

Place the vodka, lime juice, lemon juice, SomerSweet, and ice into a cocktail shaker and shake for 10 to 15 seconds, until well chilled. Strain into a martini glass and garnish with the lemon slice.

1½ ounces vodka

1 ounce freshly squeezed lime juice

Juice from ½ lemon

½ teaspoon SomerSweet (or 1 tablespoon sugar)

Ice, for shaking

Thin slice of lemon (cut across width of fruit), for garnish

Somersize Product Version

Place the vodka, margarita mix, and ice into a cocktail shaker and shake for 10 to 15 seconds, until well chilled. Strain into a martini glass and garnish with the lemon slice.

1½ ounces vodka

1½ ounces Somersize Margarita Mix

Ice, for shaking

Thin slice of lemon (cut across width of fruit), for garnish

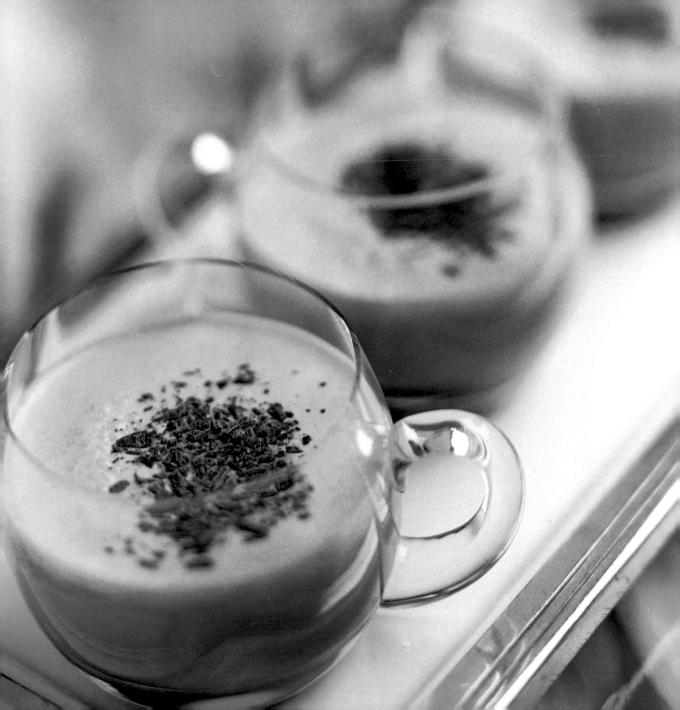

CANDY CANE HOT COCOA

SERVES 1

Here's a new way to be festive during the holidays without the added sugar: a Candy Cane Hot Cocoa. This recipe came about because of my love for Somersize Peppermint Hot Cocoa. It's so delicious! I'm giving you a recipe to make it from scratch, but the prepared mix used in the Somersize product version of this recipe is really superior.

Place the cream, cocoa, SomerSweet, and salt into a saucepan. Stir well to combine. Heat over medium until smooth. Add the mint leaves and continue stirring for 2 minutes. Strain the mint hot cocoa to remove the mint leaves and any lumps. Pour into a mug, stir in the vodka, and garnish with chocolate shavings.

Somersize Product Version

Pour Somersize Peppermint Hot Cocoa into a coffee mug with the vodka. Garnish with chocolate shavings.

2 ounces heavy cream

2 teaspoons unsweetened cocoa

1 teaspoon SomerSweet (or 1 tablespoon plus 1 teaspoon sugar)

Dash of salt

4 fresh mint leaves, coarsely chopped

1 ounce vodka

SomerSweet Dark Chocolate Shavings (or your favorite brand), for garnish

---

4 ounces prepared Somersize Peppermint Hot Cocoa

1 ounce vodka

SomerSweet Dark Chocolate Shavings, for garnish

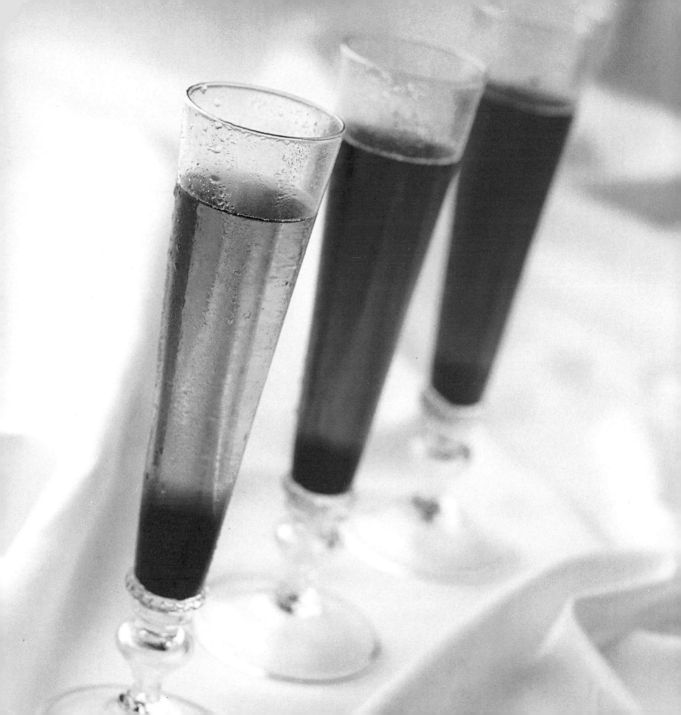

COSMOSA

SERVES 1

Sunday brunch or ladies' lunch—this drink sets just the right mood. It's pink and pretty and light. Garnish with a beautiful orchid or pink rose petals.

In a pitcher, combine the cranberry juice, lime juice, and SomerSweet until SomerSweet dissolves. Pour into a champagne flute or over ice. Add the champagne, gently stir to combine, and garnish as desired.

1½ ounces unsweetened
  cranberry juice
Juice of ½ Key lime
  (or ¼ regular Persian lime)
Squeeze of fresh lime juice
½ teaspoon SomerSweet
  (or 2 teaspoons sugar)

Somersize Product Version

Pour the ingredients into a champagne flute or over ice. Gently stir to combine and garnish as desired.

4 ounces champagne
2 ounces Somersize
  Cosmopolitan Mix

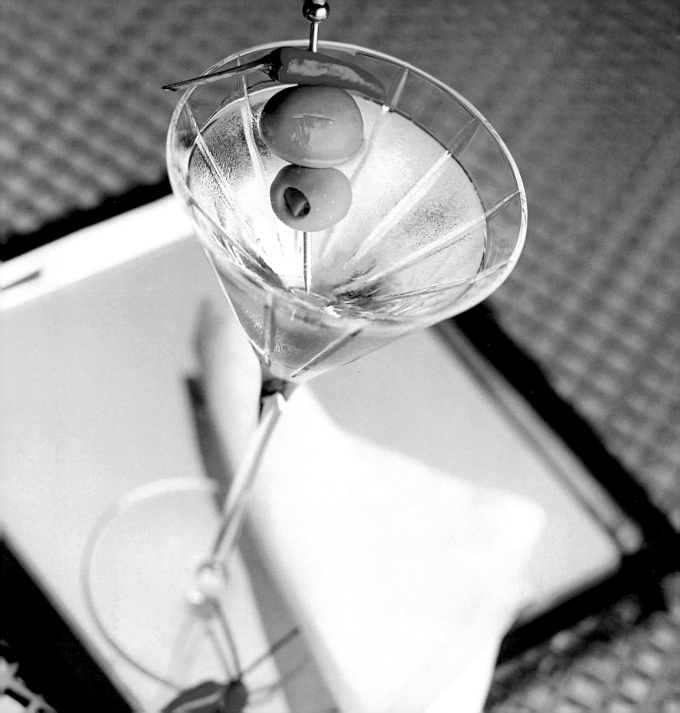

DIRTY JALAPEÑO MARTINI

SERVES 1

For those of us who only order a martini so that we can hold the glass and eat the olive, this one's for you. *Dirty* means you get a little extra olive juice, but this version adds a kick: the jalepeño-stuffed olive garnish is joined by a Thai red chili to really spice it up! You can find the red chilies in the produce section.

Break open 2 of the Thai red chili peppers to release their natural spice (capsaicin oil), and place them into a cocktail shaker with the vodka, olive juice, and ice. Shake well and strain into a chilled martini glass. Skewer the olives with the remaining red chili as a garnish.

3 small Thai red chilies

3 ounces premium vodka

1/4 ounce juice from a jar of jalapeño-stuffed olives

Ice

3 jalapeño-stuffed olives (sold in jars), for garnish

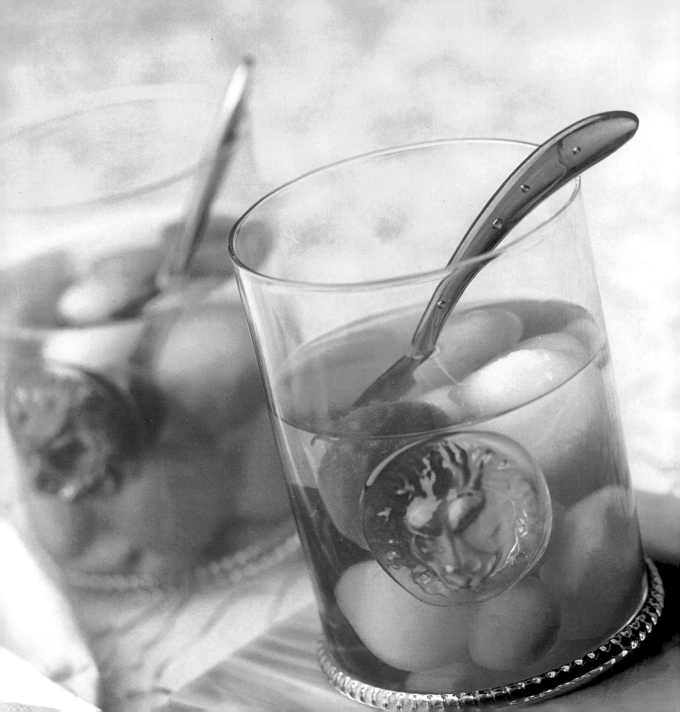

JUNGLE JUICE

SERVES 12

This is more fruit than it is a drink, but the combo is delightful. You simply marinate the fruit overnight and then enjoy it with the juice the following day. You may serve it in the watermelon bowl or place fruit and juice into glasses.

Slice the watermelon in half. Make melon balls from the flesh and set aside. Scoop out half of the watermelon to use as a bowl. Scoop out all the seeds from the other melons and make melon balls. Add all three types of melon balls with their juice to the watermelon bowl. Cut the pineapple into chunks and add them, and their juice, to the melon balls. Gently toss the melon and pineapple. Pour vodka or rum over the fruit and place in the refrigerator for about 24 hours to let the flavors meld.

Spoon the fruit into glasses with some of the juice from the bottom of the bowl.

1 watermelon, with juice
1 cantaloupe melon, with juice
1 honeydew melon, with juice
1/2 pineapple, with juice
1 pint vodka or light rum

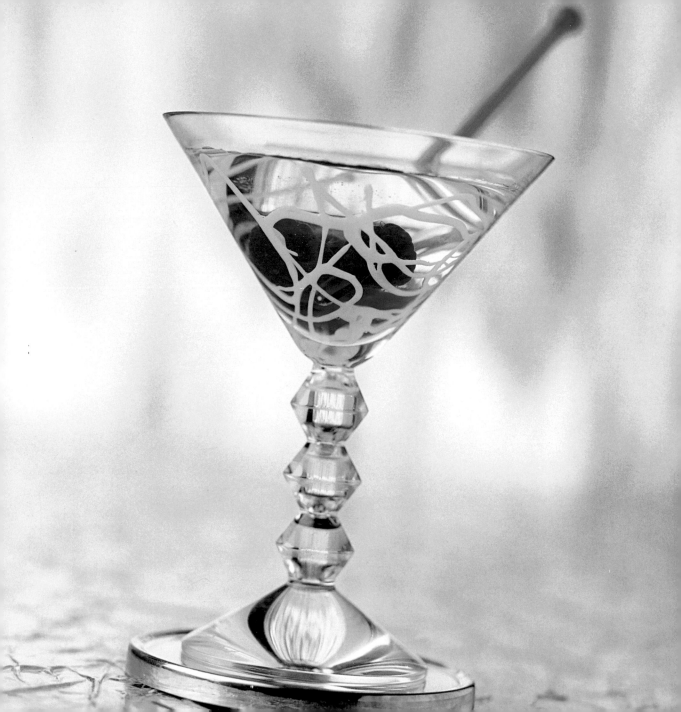

THE BERRY CHOCOLATE MARTINI

SERVES 1

Berries with chocolate is one of my favorite dessert combinations. Now it's also one of my favorite drinks! This drink has a spectacular presentation and it tastes divine. It's not overly sweet as you might expect. You simply drizzle melted chocolate into a chilled glass and the essence of the chocolate infuses with the berries to add the perfect amount of sin. A great dessert drink. I like it with white chocolate!

Using a fork, drizzle melted SomerSweet Baking Chocolate into a chilled martini glass. Drop 5 or 6 berries into the glass. Place the vodka, unsweetened cranberry juice, a few of each berry, the SomerSweet, and ice into a cocktail shaker and shake for 15 to 20 seconds to release the juice from the berries. Strain into the martini glass.

3 squares of SomerSweet
  Baking Chocolate (or your
  favorite brand), melted
5 or 6 assorted berries,
  for garnish
2 to 3 ounces premium vodka
Splash of unsweetened or
  regular cranberry juice
1/4 cup fresh berries
  (such as raspberries,
  blueberries, blackberries,
  or strawberries)
1/2 teaspoon SomerSweet

Somersize Product Version

Using a fork, drizzle melted SomerSweet Chocolate into a chilled martini glass. Drop 5 or 6 berries in the glass. Place the vodka, Somersize Cosmopolitan Mix, a few of each berry, and ice into a cocktail shaker and shake for 15 to 20 seconds to release the juice from the berries. Strain into the martini glass.

3 squares of SomerSweet
  Baking Chocolate, melted
5 to 6 assorted berries,
  for garnish
2 to 3 ounces premium vodka
Splash of Somersize
  Cosmopolitan Mix
1/4 cup of fresh berries
  (such as raspberries,
  blueberries, blackberries,
  or strawberries)

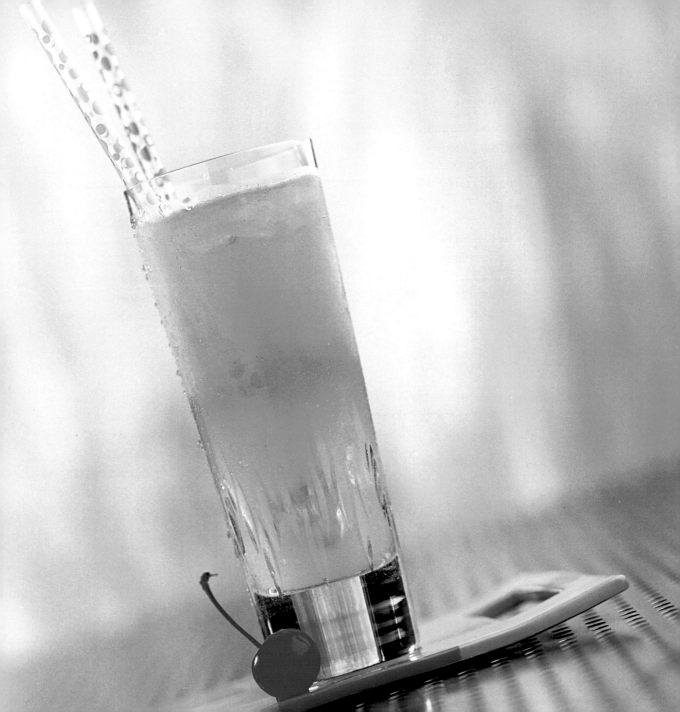

LONG ISLAND ICED TEA

SERVES 1

Grab a couple of straws and a designated driver with this one. It's tall and cool, and one is definitely enough!

Place ice into a highball glass. Add all the ingredients except the cola and the lemon wedge and stir to combine. Pour the cola onto a spoon over the drink. This keeps the cola floating on the top for a lovely presentation. Garnish with the lemon wedge.

Ice
1/2 ounce vodka
1/2 ounce 100% agave tequila
1/2 ounce light rum
1/2 ounce gin
1/2 ounce orange juice
2/3 ounce lime juice
1/3 ounce lemon juice
1/2 teaspoon SomerSweet
  (or 2 teaspoons sugar)
1/2 ounce diet, caffeine-free
  cola
1 lemon wedge, for garnish

Somersize Product Version

Place ice into a highball glass. Add all the ingredients except the cola and the lemon wedge and stir to combine. Pour the cola onto a spoon over the drink. This keeps the cola floating on the top for a lovely presentation. Garnish with the lemon wedge.

Ice
1/2 ounce vodka
1/2 ounce 100% agave tequila
1/2 ounce light rum
1/2 ounce gin
1/2 ounce orange juice
1 ounce Somersize Margarita
  Mix
1/8 teaspoon SomerSweet
  (or 1/2 teaspoon sugar)
1/2 ounce diet, caffeine-free
  cola
1 lemon wedge, for garnish

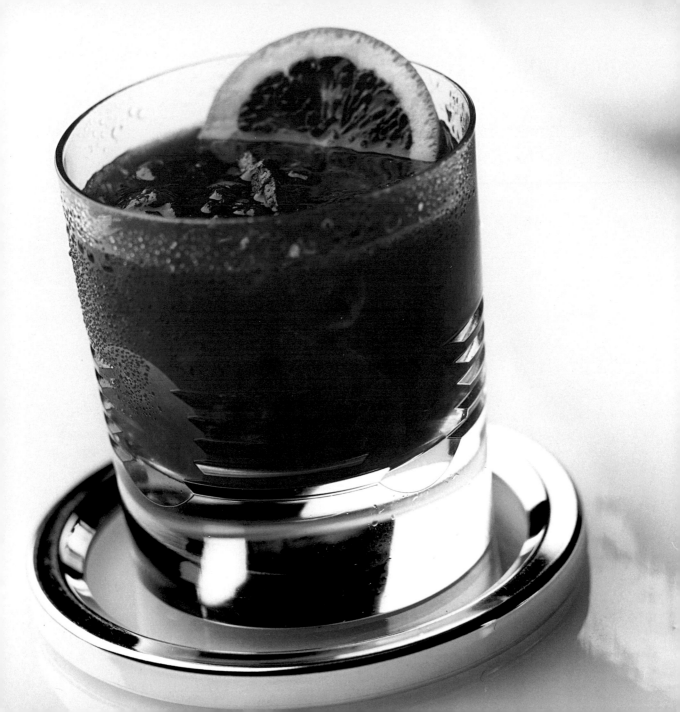

BLOOD ORANGE SCREWDRIVER

SERVES 1

This European twist on the original is an exotic brunch drink. Look for fresh blood oranges during their short season in spring, or order blood orange juice from dreamfoods.com.

Place the vodka, blood orange juice, and SomerSweet into a cocktail shaker with ice and mix thoroughly. Pour the entire contents into a highball glass and garnish with a blood orange slice.

1 1/2 ounces vodka

4 ounces blood orange juice

1/4 teaspoon SomerSweet
   (or 1 teaspoon sugar)

Ice

Blood orange slice,
   for garnish

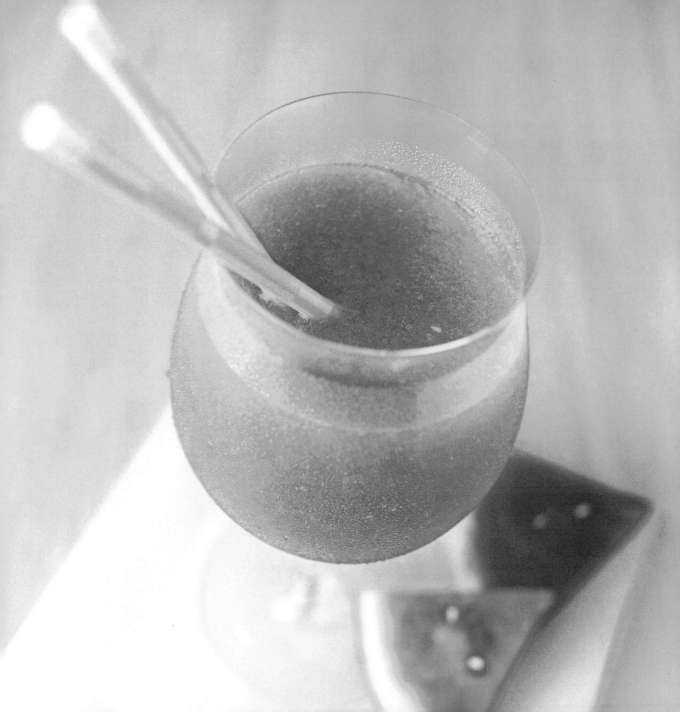

WATERMELON DAIQUIRI

SERVES 2

This drink is beautiful made with or without the alcohol. Think pink! It's best to freeze the watermelon ahead of time. If you don't have time, add ice to create a frozen creation. I prefer the frozen melon so its taste does not become diluted.

Place the frozen watermelon into a blender with the SomerSweet, lime juice, and vodka. (Add ice if the watermelon is not frozen.) Blend until smooth and serve in a margarita glass with a watermelon wedge.

1½ cups (12 ounces) seedless
  watermelon, cut into
  chunks and frozen
1 teaspoon SomerSweet
  (or 1 tablespoon plus
  1 teaspoon sugar)
Juice from ½ Key lime
  (or ¼ regular Persian lime)
1½ ounces vodka or
  light rum
Watermelon wedge,
  for garnish

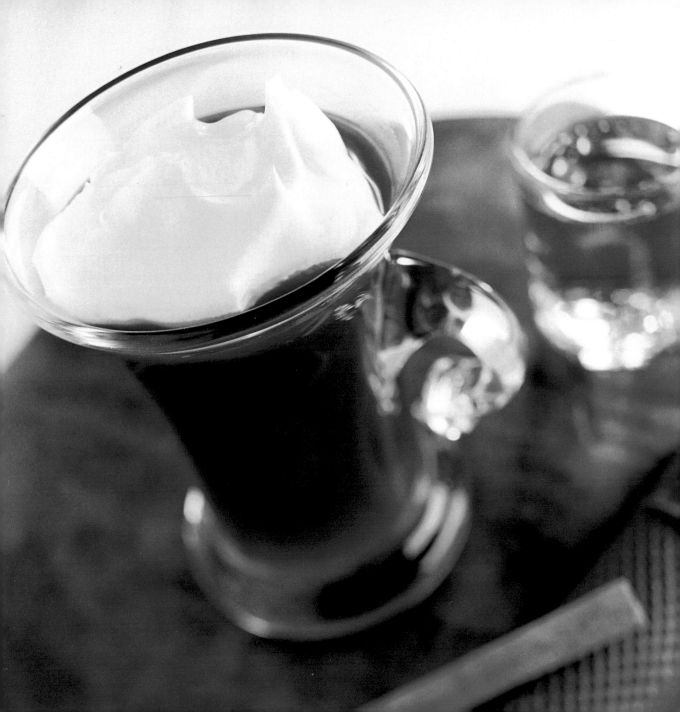

IRISH COFFEE

SERVES 1

On a cold winter night, this is a nice one to warm you up. I add a touch of mint for another layer of taste.

Prepare the garnish by pouring the cream into a mixing bowl and adding the SomerSweet. Beat the cream until it reaches a stiff whipped-cream consistency. Set aside.

   To make the coffee, place the SomerSweet and the mint leaf into the bottom of a mug. Add the coffee and the whiskey. Stir to combine. Top with a dollop of the whipped cream. Serve immediately.

FOR GARNISH
2 ounces heavy cream
$1/2$ teaspoon SomerSweet
   (or 2 teaspoons sugar)

FOR COFFEE
1 mint leaf
$1/2$ teaspoon SomerSweet
   (or 2 teaspoons sugar)
5 ounces hot, freshly brewed,
   strong decaffeinated coffee
1 ounce whiskey

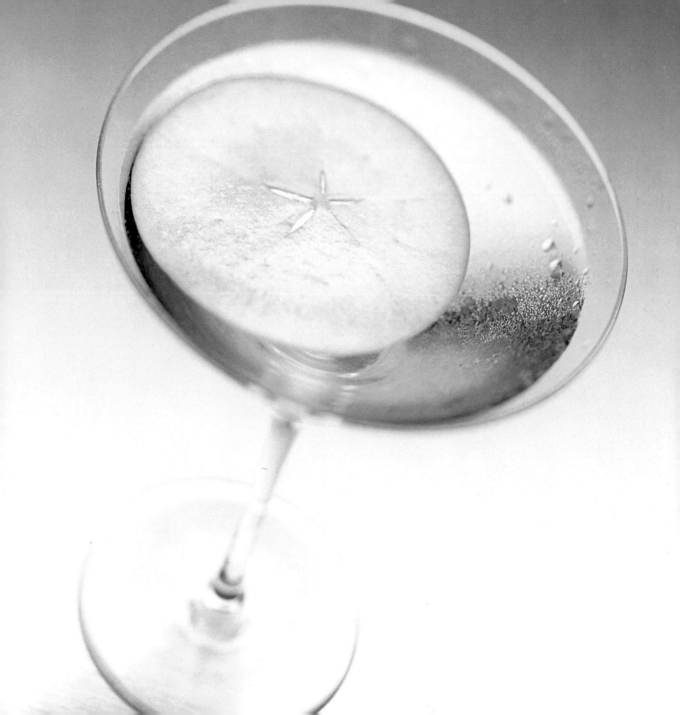

FRESH APPLE MARTINI

SERVES 1

As I mentioned earlier, I don't drink much hard alcohol, but when I had my first taste of an apple martini I just loved the tart, sweet flavor. It was like drinking candy; but who wants all that sugar? Both versions of this recipe are fabulous and neither is made with refined sugars. Use my Somersize Apple Martini Mix for a traditional "appletini" or make a fresh apple martini for a clean, crisp taste that will change your opinion of this typically candy-like drink.

Peel the apple and cut into ¼-inch cubes, avoiding the seeds. Place the apple cubes, SomerSweet and vodka in a cocktail shaker. Shake vigorously for 15 to 20 seconds to bring the juice out of the apple. Add the ice and shake again for 15 to 20 seconds to chill well. Strain into a martini glass and garnish with the apple slice.

½ Granny Smith apple
1 teaspoon SomerSweet
  (or 1 tablespoon plus
  1 teaspoon sugar)
2½ ounces premium vodka
Ice
1 thin slice of apple (cut
  across width of fruit),
  for garnish

Somersize Product Version

Place the vodka, Somersize Apple Martini Mix, and ice in a cocktail shaker. Shake vigorously for 15 to 20 seconds to chill well. Strain into a martini glass and garnish with the apple slice.

2 ounces premium vodka
1 ounce Somersize Apple
  Martini Mix
Ice
1 thin slice of apple (cut
  across width of fruit),
  for garnish

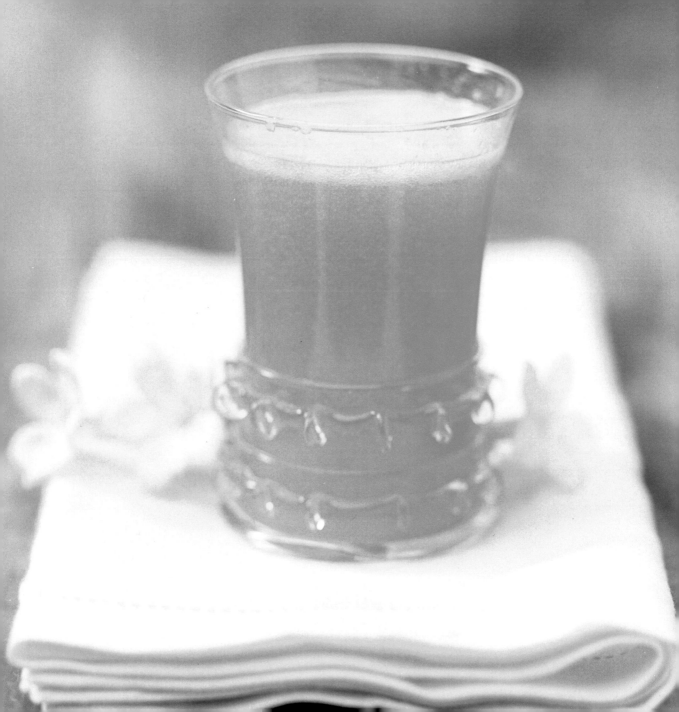

TANGERINE POMEGRANATE FIZZ

SERVES 1

This drink is like fairy nectar. Delicate, delicious, and delightful as a nonalcoholic drink, too.

Pour the vodka, tangerine juice, pomegranate juice, and SomerSweet into a cocktail shaker with ice and shake thoroughly. Add the soda water and pour the entire contents into a highball glass or old-fashioned glass and garnish as desired.

1½ ounces vodka

2 ounces tangerine juice

2 ounces unsweetened
  pomegranate juice

½ teaspoon SomerSweet
  (or 2 teaspoons sugar)

About ½ cup ice

½ ounce soda water

Tangerine slice, for garnish
  (optional)

Flowers, for garnish
  (optional)

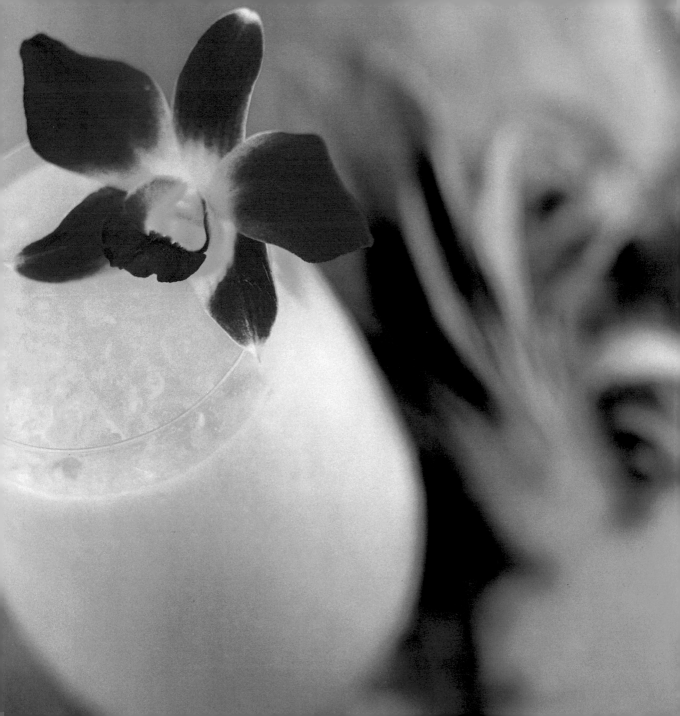

PIÑA COLADA

SERVES 2

This is the ultimate vacation drink, whether you are on an island or a cruise. Now you can have it fresh, without the serious amount of sugar you get with prepared mixers. To make it from scratch, look for unsweetened coconut milk in the ethnic section of your grocery store. It makes for a creamy, delicious drink. Or try my Somersize Piña Colada mix. Makes me want to hula.

Place all drink ingredients into a blender and blend until smooth. Divide between 2 highball glasses and garnish with a bright orchid and a pineapple wedge.

4 ounces rum
1/4 cup (2 ounces) unsweetened pineapple chunks with juice
2 ounces unsweetened coconut milk
2 teaspoons SomerSweet (or 2 1/2 tablespoons sugar)
2 cups ice
2 orchids, for garnish
2 pineapple wedges, for garnish

Somersize Product Version

Place all the drink ingredients into a blender and blend until smooth. Divide between 2 highball glasses and garnish with a bright orchid and a pineapple wedge.

4 ounces rum
8 ounces Somersize Pina Colada Mix
2 cups ice
2 orchids, for garnish
2 pineapple wedges, for garnish

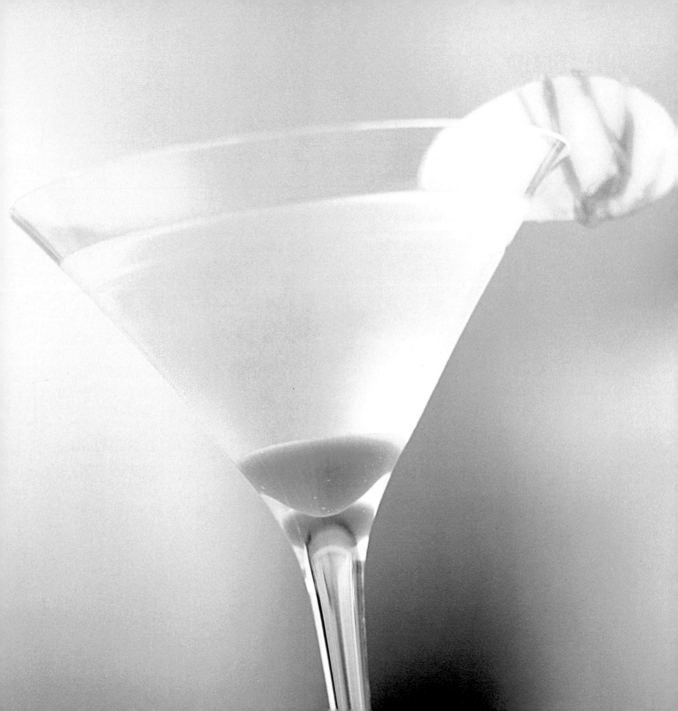

CARAMEL APPLE MARTINI

SERVES 1

If an apple martini is good, a caramel apple martini is outrageous! The caramel sauce slightly infuses the flavor of the apple martini and the result is more thrilling than a ride at Coney Island.

Warm the Somersize Hot Caramel Sauce and place a spoonful into the bottom of a chilled martini glass. Peel and cut the apple into ¼-inch cubes. Add the apple cubes, vodka, and SomerSweet to a cocktail shaker. Shake vigorously for 15 to 20 seconds to release juice from the apple. Add ice and shake again for 15 to 20 seconds to chill well. Strain into the glass and garnish with the caramel apple wedge.

Somersize Hot Caramel Sauce
  (or your favorite brand)
½ Granny Smith apple
2½ ounces premium vodka
1 teaspoon SomerSweet
  (or 1 tablespoon plus
  1 teaspoon sugar)
Ice
Apple wedge drizzled with
  caramel sauce, for garnish

Somersize Product Version

Warm the Somersize Hot Caramel Sauce and place a spoonful into the bottom of a chilled martini glass. Add the vodka, Somersize Apple Martini Mix, and ice to a cocktail shaker. Shake vigorously for 15 to 20 seconds. Strain into the glass and garnish with the caramel apple wedge.

Somersize Hot Caramel Sauce
2 ounces premium vodka
1 ounce Somersize Apple
  Martini Mix
Ice
Apple wedge drizzled with
  caramel sauce, for garnish

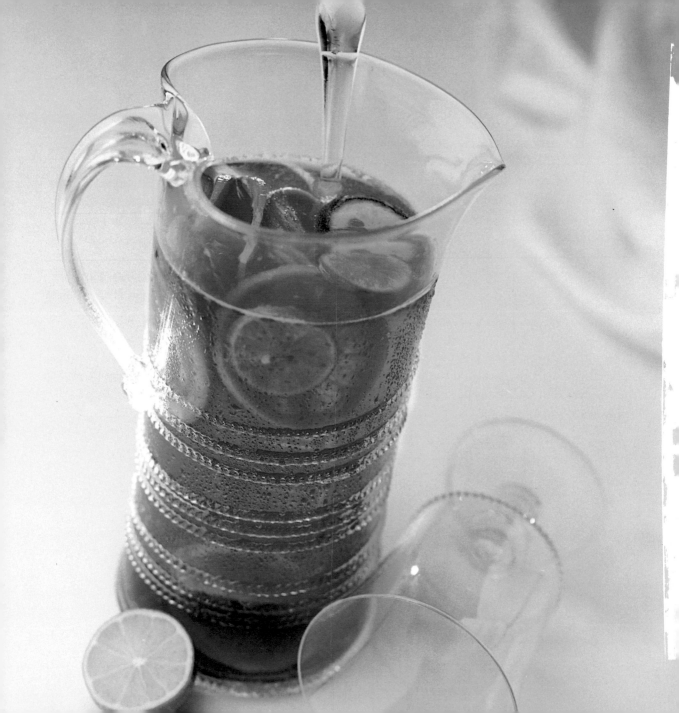

SANGRIA

SERVES 6

Sangria is a fruity, spiced wine that makes a nice daytime drink. Serve it with a Mediterranean lunch for a festive combo. No need to use your best wine here. A moderately priced bottle will do. For the best flavor, prepare 4 to 7 days in advance.

Place the wine, SomerSweet, and orange, lemon and lime juices into a large saucepan and warm over medium heat. Stir until the SomerSweet is completely dissolved. Add the squeezed fruit peels and the apple cubes. Pour into a sun-tea jar and place in the refrigerator for at least 48 hours and as long as 7 days. Add the cloves and cinnamon sticks a day before serving.

Serve with the marinated fruit for a rustic presentation or strain into a serving pitcher with fresh slices of fruit for garnish. Add a splash of soda water to each highball glass and serve over a mixture of fresh fruit garnish and ice.

1 bottle red wine

5 teaspoons SomerSweet
(or $1/2$ cup sugar)

1 cup orange juice, plus
orange peels

1 cup lemon juice, plus
lemon peels

Juice from 2 Key limes, plus
lime peels

$1/2$ Granny Smith apple,
chopped into 1-inch cubes

1 teaspoon whole cloves

1 cinnamon stick

Soda water

Thin slices of orange, lemon,
and lime (cut across width
of fruit), for garnish

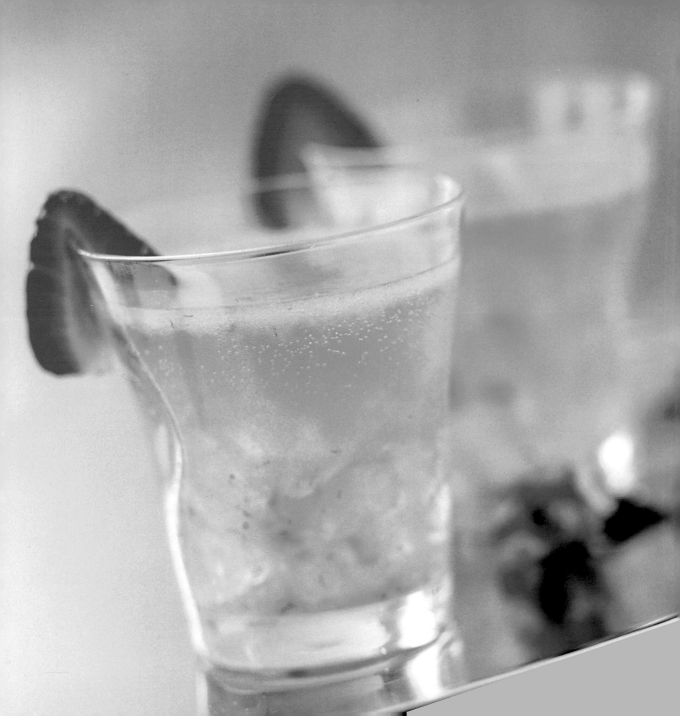

STRAWBERRY FIZZ

SERVES 1

You will want to throw a party around this drink. It's enchanting! You get little bits of fresh berries in every sip. Perfect without alcohol as well.

Remove the stems from and slice 4 or 5 of the strawberries. Place into a cocktail shaker with the vodka, SomerSweet, and ice. Shake vigorously to release the juice and fresh flavor from the strawberries. Strain into an old-fashioned glass over ice and add soda water to taste. Garnish with the whole fresh strawberry.

4 or 5 fresh strawberries,
plus one for garnish
$1^1/_2$ ounces vodka
1 teaspoon SomerSweet
(or 1 tablespoon plus
1 teaspoon sugar)
Ice
$^1/_2$ ounce soda water

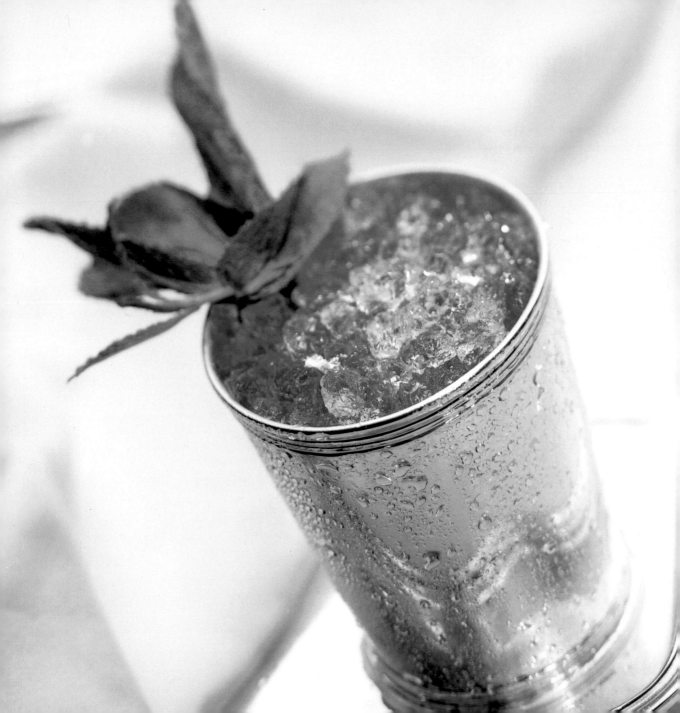

MINT JULEP

SERVES 1

There are many reasons to drink a mint julep: but the best one is so you can wear a big, fancy hat and pretend to be at the Kentucky Derby.

Place the bourbon, mint leaves, and SomerSweet in a cocktail shaker. Shake vigorously for 15 to 20 seconds to bring out the mint flavor. Add a handful of ice and shake again for 15 to 20 seconds to chill well. Fill a mint julep cup with the remaining shaved or crushed ice and strain the contents of the shaker over the ice. Top with ½ to 2 ounces water and additional shaved ice, and garnish with the mint sprig.

2½ ounces bourbon

6 to 8 fresh mint leaves

¼ teaspoon SomerSweet (or 2 teaspoons sugar)

About 1½ cups shaved or crushed ice (two large handfuls)

Mint sprig, for garnish

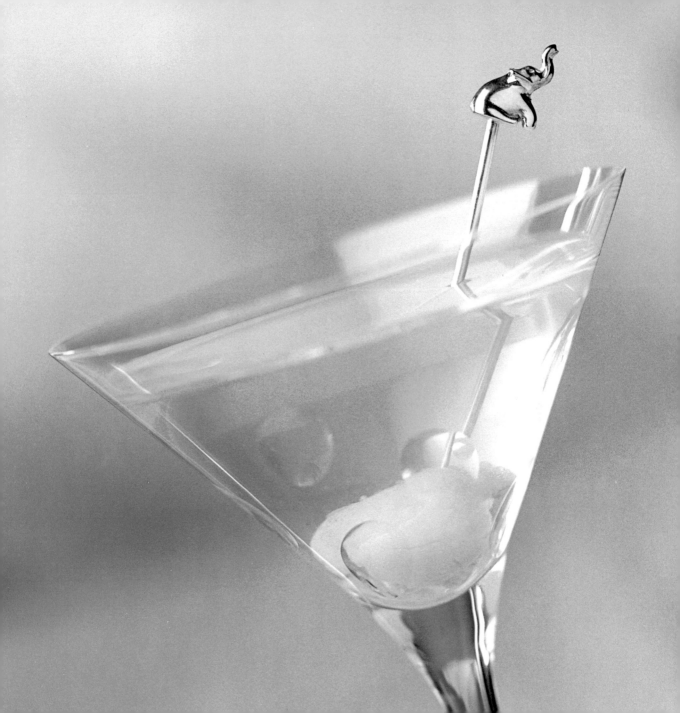

LYCHEE MARTINI

SERVES 1

I have always loved lychees, which are the plump bite-size fruit of the *Litchi chinensis* tree. Some finer Chinese restaurants serve a tray of peeled fresh lychees over ice at the end of the meal. They have a wonderful texture and an exotic perfumed flavor. Canned lychees taste different, but are also quite delicious. This martini is made with just a splash of the juice from the canned lychees and boasts a succulent lychee as a garnish. You can also buy lychee juice, which you can find at lycheesonline.com.

Place the vodka, lychee juice, SomerSweet, and ice into a cocktail shaker. Shake until well chilled. Pour into a chilled martini glass and garnish with a lychee.

$2^{1}/_{2}$ ounces premium vodka

1 ounce juice from canned lychees

$^{1}/_{4}$ teaspoon SomerSweet (or 1 teaspoon sugar)

Ice

1 lychee, fresh or canned, for garnish

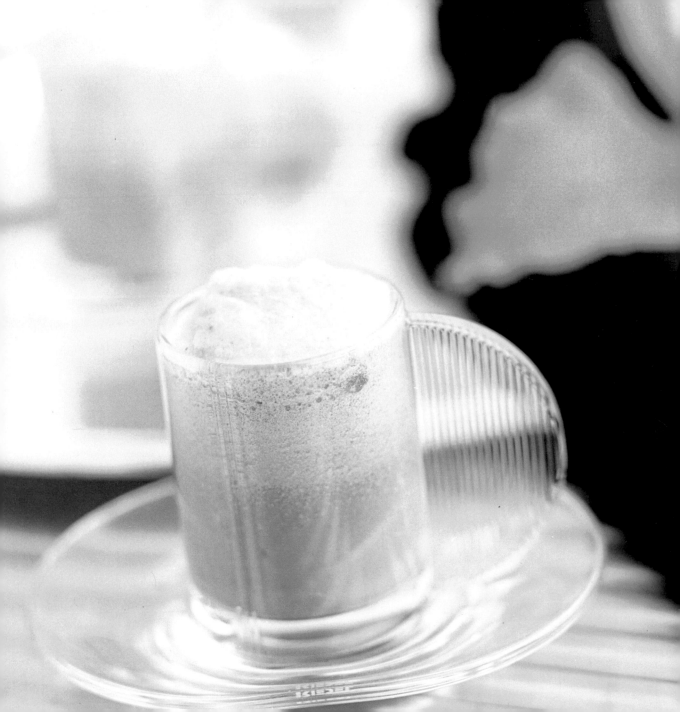

SPICED CINNAMON MOCHA

SERVES 1

In Paris they serve the most divine hot cocoa made with real cream and a touch of cinnamon. I've taken my affection for it and turned it into an after-dinner drink that will wow your guests. This is another recipe that I created because of my affection for Somersize Parisian Hot Cocoa. Usually I will tell you everything is best from scratch . . . on this one my prepared hot cocoa mix is really better! Make this to your liking with spiced rum or vodka.

Prepare the garnish by pouring the cream into a mixing bowl with the Somer-Sweet. Whip the cream until it forms stiff peaks. Set aside.

    To make the mocha, place the cocoa powder, SomerSweet, and cream into a mug. Stir well to combine. Heat in the microwave for 30 seconds, or until hot. Stir to remove any lumps. Add the hot coffee and spiced rum or vodka. Top with a dollop of the whipped cream. Sprinkle ground cinnamon on top and serve with a cinnamon stick.

Somersize Product Version

Prepare the garnish by pouring the cream into a mixing bowl with the Somer-Sweet. Whip the cream until it forms stiff peaks. Set aside.

    Mix the Somersize Parisian Hot Cocoa and the decaf coffee with spiced rum or vodka in a coffee mug. Top with a dollop of the whipped cream. Sprinkle ground cinnamon on top and serve with a cinnamon stick.

FOR GARNISH

4 ounces heavy cream

1 teaspoon SomerSweet (or 1 tablespoon plus 1 teaspoon confectioners' sugar)

FOR MOCHA

2 teaspoons unsweetened cocoa powder

1 teaspoon SomerSweet (or 1 tablespoon plus 1 teaspoon confectioners' sugar)

2 ounces heavy cream

4 ounces hot decaffeinated coffee

1½ ounces spiced rum or vodka

1 teaspoon ground cinnamon

1 cinnamon stick

FOR GARNISH

4 ounces heavy cream

1 teaspoon SomerSweet (or 1 tablespoon plus one teaspoon confectioners' sugar)

FOR MOCHA

2 ounces prepared Somersize Parisian Hot Cocoa

4 ounces hot decaffeinated coffee

1½ ounces spiced rum or vodka

1 teaspoon ground cinnamon

1 cinnamon stick

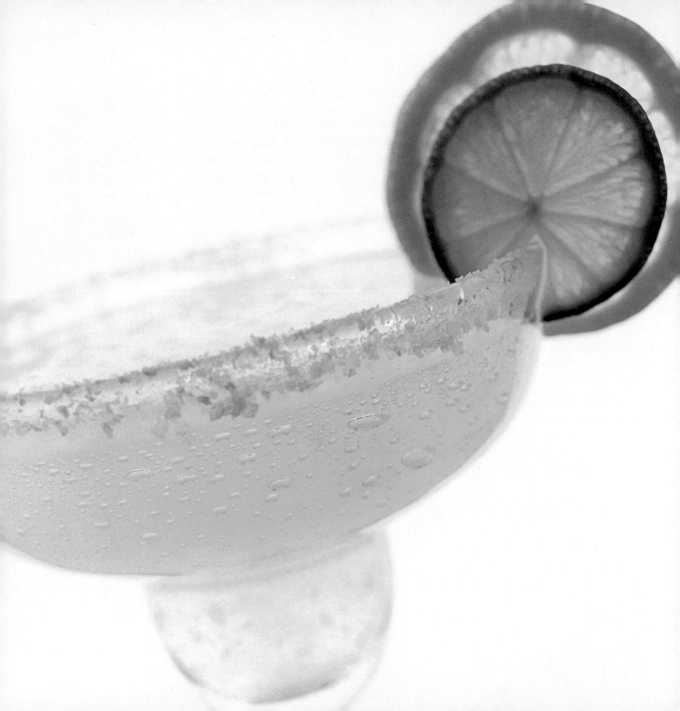

FRESH LIME MARGARITA

SERVES 2

Nothing says "fiesta" like a margarita, but most are made with sugary mixers that are filled with high fructose corn syrup. In my version, you won't miss the sugar and you'll love the fresh taste of real lime juice. Make sure to use 100 percent agave tequila, since less expensive tequilas are cut with sugar water. Or try it without alcohol for a frothy, tart blended drink.

Moisten the rims of 2 margarita glasses and dip into the salt. Place the tequila, citrus juices, SomerSweet, and ice into a blender and blend until frothy and smooth. Pour into the glasses and garnish with lemon and lime slices or spineless cactus wedges.

To serve on the rocks, shake all the drink ingredients in a cocktail shaker with ice. Pour the contents into the glasses and garnish.

Ingredients (first version):

Rimming salt for glasses (optional)

3 to 4 ounces 100% agave tequila

1 ounce orange juice

3 ounces freshly squeezed Key lime juice

Juice from 1/2 lemon

1 1/2 teaspoons SomerSweet (or 2 tablespoons sugar)

2 cups ice

Lemon and lime slices (cut across width of fruit), for garnish

Spineless cactus wedges, for garnish (optional)

Somersize Product Version

Moisten the rims of 2 margarita glasses and dip into the salt. Place the tequila, orange juice, margarita mix, and ice into a blender and blend until frothy and smooth. Pour into the glasses and garnish with lemon and lime slices or spineless cactus wedges.

To serve on the rocks, shake all the drink ingredients in a cocktail shaker with ice. Pour the contents into the glasses and garnish.

Ingredients (Somersize Product Version):

Rimming salt for glasses (optional)

3 to 4 ounces 100% agave tequila

2 tablespoons orange juice

6 ounces Somersize Margarita Mix

2 cups ice

Lemon and lime slices (cut across width of fruit), for garnish

Spineless cactus wedges, for garnish (optional)

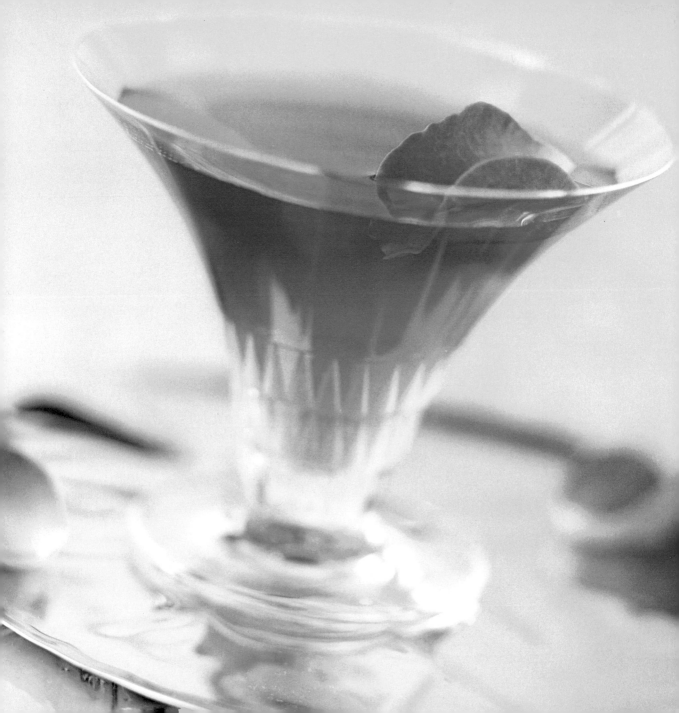

COSMOPOLITAN

SERVES 1

This pink beauty was made famous by Carrie and the girls in *Sex and the City*. Now it's in the spotlight without sugar! This is the drink I am holding on the cover, so ladies, find a piano to drape yourselves over and pour yourself a Cosmo.

Pour the vodka, juices, and SomerSweet over ice in a cocktail shaker and shake for 10 to 15 seconds. Strain into a martini glass and garnish with rose petals, an orchid or a lime wedge.

1 1/2 ounces vodka
1 1/2 ounces unsweetened
   cranberry juice
1/4 ounce orange juice
1/4 ounce lime juice
1/2 teaspoon SomerSweet
   (or 2 teaspoons sugar)
Ice
Rose petals, orchid, or lime
   wedge, for garnish

Somersize Product Version

Pour the vodka and mix over ice in a cocktail shaker and shake well. Strain into a martini glass and garnish with rose petals, an orchid, or a lime wedge.

2 ounces vodka
1 ounce Somersize
   Cosmopolitan Mix
Ice
Rose petals, orchid, or lime
   wedge, for garnish

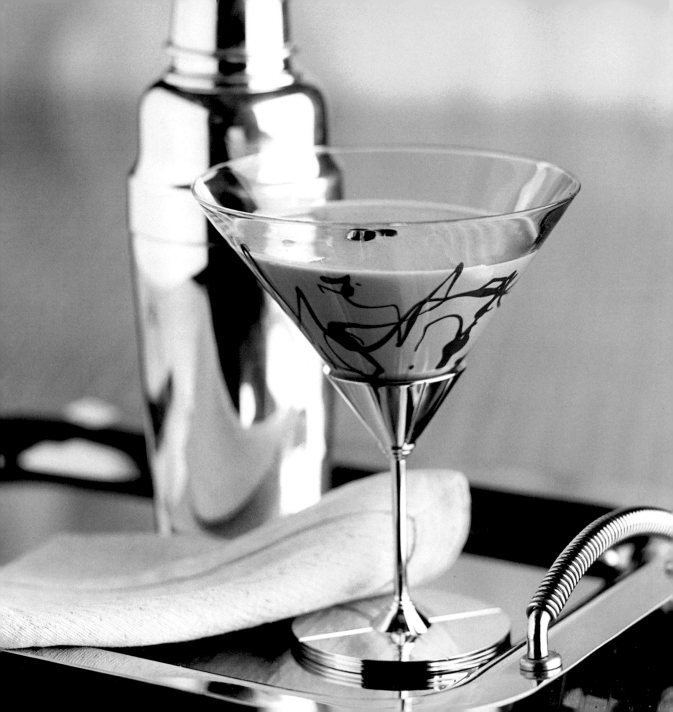

CHOCOLATE ESPRESSO MARTINI

SERVES 1

Coffee, chocolate, and cream—all shook up in a decadent martini.

Using a fork, drizzle melted SomerSweet Dark Baking Chocolate into a chilled martini glass. Mix the vodka, cream, espresso beans, espresso, Somer-Sweet, and ice in a cocktail shaker. Shake vigorously for 10 to 15 seconds. Strain into the glass and drop in dark-roasted decaffeinated espresso beans as a garnish.

3 squares SomerSweet Dark Baking Chocolate (or your favorite brand), melted

2 to 3 ounces premium vodka

1/2 ounce heavy cream

10 to 15 dark-roasted decaffeinated espresso beans

1 ounce decaffeinated espresso (or strong dark-roasted decaffeinated coffee)

1/4 teaspoon SomerSweet (or 1 teaspoon sugar)

Ice

Dark-roasted decaffeinated espresso beans, for garnish

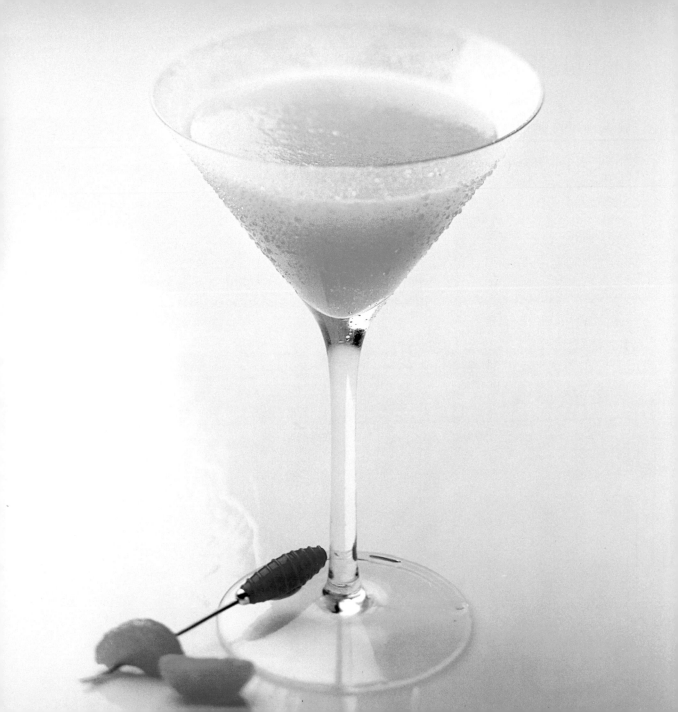

MANDARIN ORANGE MARTINI

SERVES 1

The bright color and vibrant taste of this drink will stir your senses.

Place the vodka, mandarin orange juice, mandarin orange slices, SomerSweet, and ice in a cocktail shaker. Shake vigorously to release the fresh mandarin flavor. Strain into a chilled martini glass and garnish with mandarin orange slices.

2^1/$_2$ ounces premium vodka
1 ounce unsweetened
    mandarin orange juice
15 mandarin orange slices
^{3}/$_4$ teaspoon SomerSweet
    (or 1 tablespoon sugar)
Mandarin orange slices,
    for garnish

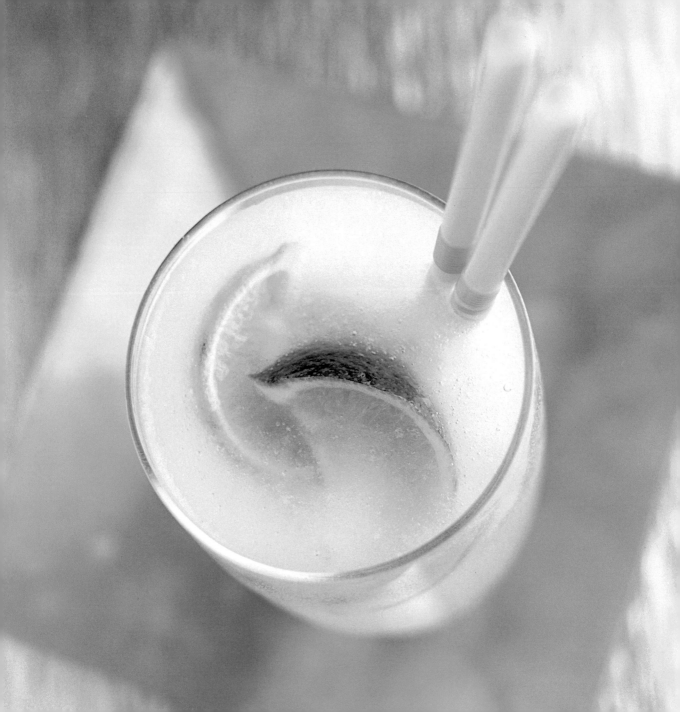

GINGER LIME COOLER

SERVES 1

This is a lovely afternoon drink, especially when you are serving Asian food. Alan loves ginger and this is one of his favorites. Without the alcohol, it becomes a perfectly tart and sweet ginger-limeade. Adjust the amount of ginger to your liking.

Place the vodka, lime juice, ginger slices, and SomerSweet into a cocktail shaker with ice and shake vigorously to release the fresh ginger flavor. Add the soda water, then pour the entire contents into a highball glass and garnish with sliced ginger and Key lime wedges.

1½ ounces vodka

Juice of 1 ½ Key limes
   (or 1 regular Persian lime)

6 to 8 thin slices peeled fresh
   ginger

1 teaspoon SomerSweet
   (or 1 tablespoon plus
   1 teaspoon sugar)

Ice

½ ounce soda water

Thin slices of peeled fresh
   ginger, for garnish

Key lime wedges, for garnish

Accessories Guide

Somersize Mojito: Imported hand-blown clear glass "Tessa 1" by Juliska, 888-414-8448, www.juliska.com. Surface by Stained Glass Supply, 2104 Colorado Blvd., Eagle Rock, CA 90041, 323-254-4361.

Mango Mojito: "Petal Cut Highball" by Steuben available with Geary's of Beverly Hills 351 North Beverly Drive, Beverly Hills, CA, 90201, 310-273-4741 or 800-793-6670, www.gearys.com. Citrus-colored glass "Bamboo" coasters by Fire and Light available at Buyers Services, 379 South Robertson, Beverly Hills, CA 90211, 310-273-8526 or 800-551-8710. Stained-glass available at Stained Glass Supply, 2104 Colorado Blvd., Eagle Rock, CA 90041, 323-254-4361.

Watermelon Mojito: "Perles" wine glass available from Lalique. For the store nearest you, call 310-271-7892 or visit www.lalique.com. Imported square (5") glass coaster available at Crate & Barrel, 75 West Colorado Blvd., Pasadena, CA 91105, 626-683-8000. For the store nearest you, call 800-323-5461 or visit www.crate-andbarrel.com. Antique glass stirrer from Suzanne's private collection.

Pomegranate Mojito: Highball by Crate & Barrel, 75 West Colorado Blvd., Pasadena, CA 91105, 626-683-8000. For the store nearest you, call 800-323-5461 or visit www.crateandbarrel.com.

Lavender Blended Citrus Smoothie: "Trumpet Flute" champagne flute available at Crate & Barrel, 75 West Colorado Blvd., Pasadena, CA 91105, 626-683-8000.

For the store nearest you, call 800-323-5461 or visit www.crateandbarrel.com. Rectangular silver tray by Christofle, 9515 Brighton Way, Beverly Hills, CA 90210, 310-858-8058, www.christofle.com. Stained-glass available at Stained Glass Supply, 2104 Colorado Blvd., Eagle Rock, CA 90041, 323-254-4361.

Ruby Red Greyhound: Imported hand-blown "Nadia 3" small glass tumbler available from Juliska, 888-414-8448, www.juliska.com.

Lemon Drop: Imported "Diamont" martini glass by Lalique. For the store nearest you, call 310-271-7892 or visit www.lalique.com. Silver tray by Ercuis Silver available at Buyers Services, 379 South Robertson, Beverly Hills, CA 90211, 310-273-8526 or 800-551-8710. Napkins from Suzanne's private collection.

Candy Cane Hot Cocoa: Glass coffee cup available at Crate & Barrel, 75 West Colorado Blvd., Pasadena, CA 91105, 626-683-8000. For the store nearest you, call 800-323-5461 or visit www.crateandbarrel.com. Pewter and ceramic tray by Arte Italica available at Buyers Services, 379 South Robertson, Beverly Hills, CA 90211, 310-273-8526 or 800-551-8710. Stained-glass surface available at Stained Glass Supply, 2104 Colorado Blvd., Eagle Rock, CA 90041, 323-254-4361.

Cosmosa: Imported hand-blown "Fiorella 2" clear champagne flute available at Juliska, 888-414-8448, www.juliska.com. Linen available at Crate & Barrel, 75 West Colorado Blvd., Pasadena, CA 91105, 626-683-

8000. For the store nearest you, call 800-323-5461 or visit www.crateandbarrel.com.

Dirty Jalapeño Martini: "Dorset" martini glass imported by Williams-Sonoma, 142 S. Lake Blvd., Pasadena, CA 91101, 626-795-5045. For store nearest you, call 800-541-1262. French silver martini picks by Ercuis Silver imported by De Vine Corporation, 732-751-0500, www.devinecorp.net. Hand-crafted "Beaten Cocktail" silver tray by Michael Aram, 866-792-2726, www.michaelaram.com. Napkins from Suzanne's private collection. Surface by Industrial Metal Supplies, 8300 San Fernando Road, Sun Valley, CA 91352, 818-729-3333.

Jungle Juice: Imported hand-blown glass "Victor Small Tumbler" by Juliska, 888-414-8448, www.juliska.com. Raw silk napkin by Ann Gish, 866-627-5800. Green glass coasters custom made with glass by Stained Glass Supply, 2104 Colorado Blvd., Eagle Rock, CA 90041, 323-254-4361. Rainbow acrylic fork available in set of eight assorted colors by Kozial available at Duck Soup at The Farmers Market/The Grove, 6333 West 3rd Street, Ste. E-16, Los Angeles, CA 90036, 310-441-8544.

The Berry Chocolate Martini: Imported "Vega" martini glass by Baccarat available at Geary's of Beverly Hills, 351 North Beverly Drive, Beverly Hills, CA 90201, 310-273-4741 or 800-793-6670, www.gearys.com. Silver-plated coaster available at Williams-Sonoma, 142 South Lake Blvd., Pasadena, CA 91101, 626-795-5045. For the store nearest you, call 800-541-1262 or visit www.williams-sonoma.com. Stirrer custom made by Stained Glass Supply, 2104 Colorado Blvd., Eagle Rock, CA 90041, 323-254-4361. All glass available at Stained Glass Supply, 2104 Colorado Blvd., Eagle Rock, CA 90041, 323-254-4361.

Long Island Iced Tea: Imported lead crystal "Duchesse" highball by Vera Wang available at Buyers Services, 379 South Robertson, Beverly Hills, CA 90211, 310-273-8526 or 800-551-8710. Ceramic "Flat-Handled Tray" (set of three) in mixed citrus block by Studio B by Magenta available at Salutations, 11640 San Vicente Blvd., Los Angeles, CA 90049, 310-820-6127. Straws by Crate & Barrel, 75 West Colorado Blvd., Pasadena, CA 91105, 626-683-8000. For the store nearest you, call 800-323-5461 or visit www.crateandbarrel.com. Surface by Industrial Metal Supplies, 8300 San Fernando Road, Sun Valley, CA 91352, 818-729-3333. Glass by Stained Glass Supply, 2104 Colorado Blvd., Eagle Rock, CA 90041, 323-254-4361.

Blood Orange Screwdriver: "Atalante" double old-fashioned glass by Christofle, 9515 Brighton Way, Beverly Hills, CA 90210, 310-858-8058, www.christofle.com. "Bell Shiny" silver metal ice bucket available at Crate & Barrel, 75 West Colorado Blvd., Pasadena, CA 91105, 626-683-8000. For the store nearest you, call 800-323-5461 or visit www.crateandbarrel.com. Silver and glass wine coaster (set of two) available at Buyers Services, 379 South Robertson, Beverly Hills, CA 90211, 310-273-8526 or 800-551-8710. Stained-glass surface available at Stained Glass Supply, 2104 Colorado Blvd., Eagle Rock, CA 90041, 323-254-4361.

Watermelon Daiquiri: Imported Austrian "Sommelier Burgundy Grand Cru" by Riedel. For the store nearest you, call 732-346-8960 or visit www.riedel.com. Imported French "Ceris Seraie" towel by Le Jacquard Francais available at Salutations, 900 Granite Drive, Pasadena, CA 91101, 626-577-7460. Straws available at Crate & Barrel, 75 West Colorado Blvd., Pasadena, CA 91105, 626-683-8000. For the store nearest you, call 800-323-5461 or visit www.crateandbarrel.com. Custom stained-glass coasters and glass available at Stained Glass Supply, 2104 Colorado Blvd., Eagle Rock, CA 90041, 323-254-4361.

Irish Coffee: Hand-blown "Irish Coffee Mug" imported from Ireland by Simon Pearce available at Geary's of Beverly Hills, 351 North Beverly Drive, Beverly Hills, CA 90201, 310-273-4741 or 800-793-6670, www.gearys.com. "Measure Shot Glass" available at Williams-Sonoma, 142 South Lake, Pasadena, CA 91101, 626-795-5045. Antique cutting board and vintage spice grater from Suzanne's private collection.

Fresh Apple Martini: Imported "Balaton" martini glass available at Crate & Barrel, 75 West Colorado Blvd., Pasadena, CA 91105, 626-683-8000. For the store nearest you, call 800-323-5461 or visit www.crate-andbarrel.com. Surface by Stained Glass Supply, 2104 Colorado Blvd., Eagle Rock, CA 90041, 323-254-4361.

Tangerine Pomegranate Fizz: Imported hand-blown "Harriet 4" by Juliska , 888-414-8448, www.juliska.com. Linen napkins available at Crate & Barrel, 75 West Colorado Blvd., Pasadena, CA 91105, 626-683-8000. For the store nearest you, call 800-323-5461 or visit www.crateandbarrel.com.

Piña Colada: Imported 20-ounce goblet available at Crate & Barrel, 75 West Colorado Blvd., Pasadena, CA 91105, 626-683-8000. For the store nearest you, call 800-323-5461 or visit www.crateandbarrel.com. Surface by Stained Glass Supply, 2104 Colorado Blvd., Eagle Rock, CA 90041, 323-254-4361.

Caramel Apple Martini: "Calloway" martini glass by Christofle, 9515 Brighton Way, Beverly Hills, CA 90210, 310-858-8058, www.christofle.com.

Sangria: Imported hand-blown glass "Fiorella 4" medium goblet and "Ella" pitcher available from Juliska, 888-414-8448, www.juliska.com. Glass martini stirrer available at Crate & Barrel, 75 West Colorado Blvd., Pasadena, CA 91105, 626-683-8000. For the store nearest you, call 800-333-5461 or visit www.crate-andbarrel.com.

Strawberry Fizz: Antique glasses from Suzanne's private collection. Hand-crafted silver "Lily Platter" by Michael Aram, 866-792-2726, www.michaelaram.com.

Mint Julep: Silver mint julep cup made in America by Lunt and available exclusively at Geary's of Beverly Hills, 351 North Beverly Drive, Beverly Hills, CA 90201, 310-273-4741 or 800-793-6670, www.gearys.com. Square silver tray by Christofle, 9515 Brighton Way, Beverly Hills, CA 90210, 310-858-8058, www.christofle.com. Imported French linen from Suzanne's private collection.

Lychee Martini: Imported "Cluny" martini glass by Christofle, 9515 Brighton Way, Beverly Hills, CA 90210, 310-858-8058, www.christofle.com. French silver "Elephant Martini Picks" by Ercuis Silver imported by De Vine, 732-751-0500, www.devinecorp.net.

Spiced Cinnamon Mocha: Imported Austrian "Espresso Cup and Saucer" by Riedel. For the store nearest you, call 732-346-8960 or visit www.riedel.com. Round silver tray by Christofle, 9515 Brighton Way, Beverly Hills, CA 90210, 310-858-8058, www.christofle.com. Imported raw silk napkin by Ann Gish, 866-627-5800.

Fresh Lime Margarita: "Warped Glass" margarita glass available at Pottery Barn, 1 East Colorado Blvd., Pasadena, CA 91105, 626-577-1474. For the store nearest you, call 888-779-5176 or visit www.potterybarn.com.

Cosmopolitan: Imported "Bourgueil" champagne coupe by Lalique. For the store nearest you, call 310-271-7892 or visit www.lalique.com. Hand-crafted silver "Lily Pad Coaster" available from Michael Aram, 866-792-2726, www.michealaram.com.

Chocolate Espresso Martini: "Challis" martini glass by Vera Wang available at Geary's of Beverly Hills, 351 North Beverly Drive, Beverly Hills, CA 90210, 800-793-6670, www.gearys.com. Silver martini shaker available at Christofle, 9515 Brighton Way, Beverly Hills, CA 90210, 310-858-8058, www.christofle.com. Italian silver tray by Stella available at Casa E Cucina Francesca, 360-563-9440. Hem-stitched "Cara Mia" yellow napkin by Vietri available at Bo Danica, 7722 Girard Avenue, La Jolla, CA 92037, 858-454-6107.

Mandarin Orange Martini: Imported "Balaton" large martini glass available at Crate & Barrel, 75 West Colorado Blvd., Pasadena, CA 91105, 626-683-8000. For the store nearest you, call 800-323-5461 or visit www.crateandbarrel.com. Surface by Stained Glass Supply, 2104 Colorado Blvd., Eagle Rock, CA 90041, 323-254-4361.

Ginger Lime Cooler: Imported glass "Bormi" tumbler available at Maison Midi, 148 South La Brea, Los Angeles, CA 90036, 323-935-3157. Composite 7-inch turquoise "Capiz" plate imported by Asiaphile available at Zero Minus Plus, 500 Broadway, Santa Monica, CA 90401, 310-395-5718. For the store nearest you, call 866-550-8325. Surface by Industrial Metal Supplies, 8300 San Fernando Road, Sun Valley, CA 91352, 818-729-3333.

Index

Apple Martini, Caramel, 55
Apple Martini, Fresh, 49

The Berry Chocolate Martini, 39
Blood Orange Screwdriver, 43

Candy Cane Hot Cocoa, 31
Caramel Apple Martini, 55
Chocolate
    Candy Cane Hot Cocoa, 31
    Espresso Martini, 71
    Martini, The Berry, 39
    Spiced Cinnamon Mocha, 65
Cocktails
    alcohol for, 11
    bar tools for, 11
    garnishes for, 12
    glasses for, 11
    pairing with appetizers, 12
Coffee
    Chocolate Espresso Martini, 71
    Irish, 47
    Spiced Cinnamon Mocha, 65
Cosmopolitan, 69

Cosmosa, 33
Cranberry juice
    Cosmopolitan, 69
    Cosmosa, 33

Daiquiri, Watermelon, 45
Dirty Jalapeño Martini, 35

Ginger Lime Cooler, 75
Grapefruit juice
    Blended Citrus Lavender Smoothie, 25
    Ruby Red Greyhound, 27

Iced Tea, Long Island, 41
Irish Coffee, 47

Jalapeño Martini, Dirty, 35
Jungle Juice, 37

Lavender Blended Citrus Smoothie, 25
Lemon Drop, 29
Lime(s)
    Blended Citrus Lavender Smoothie, 25
    Cooler, Ginger, 75
    Cosmosa, 33
    Margarita, Fresh, 67
    Pomegranate Mojito, 23
    Somersize Mojito, 17

Watermelon Daiquiri, 45
Watermelon Mojito, 21
Long Island Iced Tea, 41
Lychee Martini, 63

Mandarin Orange Martini, 73
Mango Mojito, 19
Margarita, Fresh Lime, 67
Martinis
    The Berry Chocolate, 39
    Caramel Apple, 55
    Chocolate Espresso, 71
    Dirty Jalapeño, 35
    Fresh Apple, 49
    Lychee, 63
    Mandarin Orange, 73
Mint
    Candy Cane Hot Cocoa, 31
    Julep, 61
    Mango Mojito, 19
    Pomegranate Mojito, 23
    Somersize Mojito, 17
    Watermelon Mojito, 21
Mojitos
    Mango, 19
    Pomegranate, 23
    preparing, 12
    Somersize, 17
    Watermelon, 21

Orange(s)
    Blended Citrus Lavender Smoothie, 25
    Blood, Screwdriver, 43
    Mandarin, Martini, 73
    Sangria, 57
    Tangerine Pomegranate Fizz, 51

Piña Colada, 53
Pineapple juice
    Jungle Juice, 37
    Piña Colada, 53
Pomegranate Mojito, 23
Pomegranate Tangerine Fizz, 51

Ruby Red Greyhound, 27

Sangria, 57
Screwdriver, Blood Orange, 43
Spiced Cinnamon Mocha, 65
Strawberry Fizz, 59

Tangerine Pomegranate Fizz, 51
Tequila, agave, about, 11

Watermelon
    Daiquiri, 45
    Jungle Juice, 37
    Mojito, 21